Venus Juice

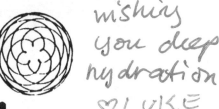

wishing
you deep
hydration
♡ LUKE

Luke Simon

Published with Numinous Books.

Cover design by Justin Sloane

Drawings by Daniel Long

Interior layout by Chriswilliamsdesign.co.uk

Author photo by Christian Defonte

ISBN: 978-1-7354710-9-9

www.the-numinous.com

To anyone who is still figuring it out,
and to the plants who give us herbs, food and flowers.

Memory is mercurial. Remembering is different then being there, and it's hard to prove if the memory is true or fiction. In my storytelling I have changed names and blended or enhanced details to play with the saturation to communicate the feelings of when I lived in L.A. April 2017- August 2018. The parts that seem the most hyperbolic are probably true.

Contents

1

Love at First Swipe

I had joked I wanted to meet my husband on Instagram, and then it actually happened. Words cast spells, and even the internet responds to magic.

I had moved Upstate to re-connect to Nature after eight years in New York City. I rented a cabin near Woodstock. Every afternoon I walked the dirt road down to the river. No one was ever there so I'd strip and mermaid in the cool water. The pure mountain water was energetically cleansing. Afterwards, I laid naked on a rock to soak up the Sun. Being naked by the river made me feel primal and free. It turned me on. The sound of the water gushing seduced me to get back in. The river current pushing my thighs, I jacked off, sending out a Love spell to my dream partner, wherever he was.

It's hard to know which Love spell worked because I did so many. I wished for Love on every frothy cappucinno heart. And I learned that in Feng Shui having pairs of things prepares your life for a partner, so I grocery shopped for veggies in twos. I arranged a still life on my kitchen counter with two peaches and two eggplants. But the spell at the river must have worked because soon after I found him.

Every night in the dark cabin I'd pour into the phone screen, hunting for Love. They say it's a numbers game, and you just have to file through enough people to find a match. But what happened that night was an algorithmic miracle. The crickets and frogs were humming loudly. The room was dark except for a flickering taper candle. I had been at the kitchen table since finishing my zucchini and eggplant stir fry, scrolling. He appeared in my discover grid: long hair up in a bun, sitting in a reading chair. His thighs were spread wide— not too skinny, not too thick, but just right. He was ironically smirking like he was annoyed to have his photo taken. He had mis-matched tattoos all over, a pixelated cherub, a sword, a calla lily. Maybe pheromones fly through Wi-Fi because my body was waking up, getting stronger for him. I sent him a message: "Hey, digging your vibe, I'm Luke." He replied immediately, "Thanks I like yours too. I'm Pablo." My energy glittered like light on water. I hadn't thought he would respond, but we texted for hours. I felt high the whole time. That was the beginning of an online friendship that grew, message by message, nude by nude, over the next few months.

Joseph Campbell said, "Leap and the net will appear." I had moved Upstate to be free and find my true calling, but so far I was just free falling, waiting for my net. I had helped establish Maha Rose Center for Healing in Brooklyn, where I offered healing sessions, but I was in a period of healing myself. There was a leak in my heart I had to fix. Because even when I focused on my accomplishments and happy memories, it always felt like something was wrong. I was trying every healing path to try to understand life and myself. Especially at night; when I was alone I felt invisible and un-formed.

Perhaps I needed to find my true calling. I studied what other healers did to market themselves, but I didn't feel confident enough in any one thing to create a brand for myself the way they did. I wanted my brand to be about not having a brand. Why do we have to be "something"? Isn't it enough to just be? I wanted to be able to drift through life, braving the unknown. But I was scared I wouldn't be able to make money as a healer and artist. I had lucid moments, but other times I felt like a bug stuck in a web, confused by my own tangled thoughts. In my cabin Upstate, I was constantly meditating, doing yoga and breathwork, clearing the energy any way I knew how, trying to get clarity on my path.

The only thing that had any clear direction in my life was Pablo. Whenever he texted, my mood and outlook changed completely. "I wish you were here," he wrote. I went out to the porch to text him under the stars. "Me too," I wrote back.

Every time he texted joy and lust rushed through me, revitalizing me. We were falling into an innovative, cloud-based version of Love.

I got to know him through the photos he posted on Instagram. His paintings were like grunge, gay Matisse. Every part of his life was touched by his creativity; he posted photos of his apartment with stacks of books, a fireplace and a Japanese monkey mask on the wall. But my favorite photos were of his face. He had long, kind eyes and thick lips, with pencil strokes of a mustache coming in. He looked like the child of Bugs Bunny and Keanu Reeves. He was everything I wanted to be: an artist, playful and confident. He always cracked a mischievous smile in the nude photos he sent me, in front of the mirror of his art studio, wearing nothing but his red Adidas sandals. In our texts I learned that he had been a sex worker, and we talked about shadow work and healing. He wanted to live brighter and was inspired by my spiritual path. I'd finally met the yang to my yin. I went to bed imagining what his touch would be like.

After talking for a few months I wanted to meet in real life. He lived in Portland and I offered to buy him a ticket to New York using miles, but his response was murky, a maybe. He used to respond right away, but now it was a casual few days later. "Sorry I was painting." The cabin was getting colder every night. "How's Portland?" I texted him, and waited to see the animated ellipsis of him responding ... But he wasn't there. I tried to read an astrology book by candlelight, checking my phone at the end of every paragraph. Maybe I could decode my destiny through the stars. I needed to figure out what would make me feel alive, besides guys. I wanted to be horny for life, not just for him. Why wasn't he responding? I blew out my candelabra and went to bed.

After the leaves fell it got too cold for swimming and hiking. I had been Upstate for six months and my dream of existing in peace in Nature hadn't panned out. The cabin felt pressurized with my emotions. I felt more lost than ever. I sat at the kitchen table with a fresh cup of chai and did my morning journaling. The word dump helped me get out my worries: how do I make money in a way that feels fulfilling? The skeletal trees stretched towards the Sun out the window. What I really wanted was to live poetically and translate life's ephemeral beauty into form. But what form? I still wasn't sure. I didn't want to work a normal job, but I couldn't grasp what I was meant to do. The house creaked and shifted in the cold. I remembered a therapist saying, "Wherever you go, there you are." Even though I had escaped to Nature, here I was, the same lost feeling had returned. The problem wasn't the place, it was me. Or was the problem the world? In a broken system, isn't failure actually a sign of success? I needed help.

I had heard of life coach Dana Balicki through friends in the healing community. She has hazel wolf eyes, shaggy hair and posts about her dream life in Joshua Tree. Dana had figured out how to be a healer who wasn't cookie cutter, but had a clear offering people could grab onto. Her program wasn't about productivity exercises, but about uncovering what you really wanted. I had been considering the program for a few weeks, but I was stuck on the money. I imagined all the clothes I could buy with this chunk of money (not to mention two months' rent). It is hard to splurge on non-physical luxuries. They exist on a subtler level. But was that the layer of my life that was depleted, empty? The part I needed to learn to fill? To heal? I had been devoted to healing for so long because I needed it so bad. I clicked around Dana's website. It had watercolor backgrounds, testimonials, and photos of her in flared jeans. She got life. She had what I wanted: an authentic career that was a natural expression of who you are. She offered a payment plan and I decided to do it. If it worked, it would be a priceless investment.

The next Tuesday, I spread a floral quilt on the floor and pulled the landline over with its curly cord. During our first session I told her how confused I was about where to head in life, if I was supposed to be a healer or an artist. She responded, "Confusion itself is a choice, and maybe a comfortable one for you." I wrote that down in my journal to consider later.

Every week Dana would guide me in creating affirmations and visualizations to influence my subconscious. "We are renovating your inner world, looking at the way you think about yourself so you can create new patterns," she'd told me.

"Okay my dear, so how do you want your life to feel? Just allow whatever words or images want to emerge." Winter rain was smacking the cabin windows, but I closed my eyes and focused. I envisioned myself with a guy, driving through a canyon by the ocean. We were both wearing shorts and he was my partner. He reached over and put his hand on my thigh as we cruised through the Sun glowing on the yellow grass of the hills.

"Did you get a visual?" Dana asked.

"Yes," I said, still basking in the feeling.

"Now just see what words come as an affirmation you can use to remind yourself of this feeling."

"My life is fabulously fulfilling," I said.

"Perfect!" Dana replied. "It's about changing the way you see yourself and the story you tell yourself. Healing from victimhood into empowerment. Personal power is knowing your truth and designing your life around it." I jotted this all down in my notebook.

I had already been experimenting with manifestation. Was a life path carved through willpower or destiny? Do our thoughts really influence our reality? I wanted to believe it was as simple as thinking positively, but I was skeptical. It couldn't be that easy. But Dana introduced me to an important missing step; clearing limiting beliefs that block you from what you want. Dana's emphasis on facing the resistance made better sense. The message of "good vibes only" had created a schism in me. What was I supposed to do with all my other vibes? When the words came to me—I wish for my life to be fabulously fulfilling—I realized I had been stuck in the opposite. I was used to seeing my life as not being good enough yet. Because I chronically thought my life wasn't good enough, I made decisions that led me to experience, or magically manifest, this blocking belief. Dana was the guide I needed. She did what a healer does: not just wave a wand, but hold your hand, create a space where you can realize how you can heal yourself. "You've been seeing the world through shit-colored lenses," Dana said. "It's not about making your lenses rose-colored, but about making your vision clear."

In week three we started working on my Inner Child. When I imagined my child self, he was waiting for someone, holding a Barbie, feeling alone. I told Dana about how much I loved Barbies and Madonna when I was little. I learned to keep it a secret, and pose as a "normal boy" so I wouldn't make people uncomfortable. Dana listened and I started to cry as I told her. "It sounds like you learned from a young age that it wasn't safe for you to be yourself," she said. I had mostly avoided those memories, had kept them hidden like the dolls in my drawer. Alone, in silence, was the only place I could finally be myself. I saw in that session with Dana how doubt and lostness had been echoing ever since. This is what I wanted to heal from. "So, let's start by forgiving that little boy who had desires and was told they were wrong," Dana said. "Maybe your confusion goes back to being unsure if it's safe to be yourself. Your inner voice is still there, it's still strong, you just have to allow it." I wouldn't have been able to go there without Dana. Sometimes you need somebody to hold your hand and guide you into the places you've learned to avoid.

"What's the price of not hearing your inner voice?" she asked.

"Sadness, frustration, no fun," I said.

I remembered the rapture of dancing to Madonna's "Cherish" music video when I was four. It had both mermaids *and* Madonna. I wanted to feel that innocent joy again. *The Little Mermaid* had just come out and I had an Ariel doll with red hair and a metallic green tail. Even at age four, I related to the Little Mermaid's longing to be part of another world where you could be yourself. I knew New York was where I could belong as a freak. Eventually, I made it, but childhood wounds take time and work to heal. I was free to be a freak in New York, but inwardly couldn't let myself. "I hear my inner voice," was the affirmation we came up with. After the session I felt light and fluid. Facing and naming that emotional scar, brought awareness and clarity. I was ready to taking my Barbies out of the inner drawers, to find my way back to that same joy and express it rather then hide it.

Pablo and I planned our first meeting for New Year's Eve in Los Angeles. I would be visiting my family in New Mexico and would drive to Cali after the holidays. My friend Marie joined me. When our car rental was upgraded from a compact to a black Mustang convertible, we agreed it was a sign that we were in Divine flow. The sunset was like melting sherbet as we headed West. I sped through the night in the Mustang, wired by the excitement and nerves of seizing my destiny.

"Is this it?" We had reached a cul-de-sac looking for Marie's friend's house.

"I don't know I've never been here, lol," Marie said.

It was 4am and all the houses were dark, everyone sleeping. Marie rolled down her window—"look, see that skeleton hanging in the tree? That's her vibe. This must be it."

The silky night air came into the car. I U-turned to find parking but scraped the curb. "*Scheisse!*" Dogs started to bark and lights turned on in the windows. We parked at a meter on the main street. Walking back up the hill I was enchanted by the thick, still air. The flowers were awake, exhaling their night-time fragrance. LA is full of flowers, and that they exist amongst such a sprawling and polluted city makes them seem even more miraculous and precious. It was hard to quit smelling them, but we were exhausted and went upstairs to Marie's friend's music room she was letting us crash in.

At 8am we went to pay the parking meter and inspect the scratch on the fender. I was screwed. I hadn't bought insurance so getting the car repainted would be expensive. Marie rubbed the place where the metal was showing through. "Let's just get some nail polish or a marker, it's not that bad," she said.

"This is why I hang out with geniuses," I said.

She pulled a Sharpie from her bag and scribbled over the gash. It healed like magic. Maybe we weren't out of the flow after all. We had parked by the Mexican Consulate and now there were women with tamale and juice carts. It was the perfect breakfast: pork tamales and nopal, spinach and orange juice. Washing the cornmeal down with tangy sweet juice I was grateful to be alive for another day.

At noon I texted Pablo: "Hey I got to LA, you here yet?"

One hour waiting for him to reply turned into another.

I didn't want to make any other plans because I wanted to be free to hang out with him. But I needed a distraction, so at noon I went to a vintage shop. I dug through a bin of silk scarves, grandma sunglasses and trucker caps, but he was still my focus. I looked up from my digging when anyone entered the shop door—maybe it would be him and this is how we were destined to meet, coincidentally, in this dusty shop.

Every time I heard my phone ding with a new text I was flooded with hope. But it was just my parents making sure I'd made it safely to LA. Then another ding—an automated follow up to rate the car rental company's customer service. I always give five stars; why not spread the Love and create some positive karma?

I went from the men's workwear section to the sequined evening gown section. I wanted to make a strong impression for our first meeting. He opened up new possibilities; I could become someone new. I filed through hangers, not even looking, too distracted by my ruminating over why he wasn't texting back. What if I didn't get to take his long hair down from his bun? What if we didn't meet and kiss at midnight? The only thing I liked at the shop was a pair of sparkly jelly platform sandals, but they weren't my size.

On the street I checked Instagram. He had posted a photo with the caption: "Cali bound ..." My heartbeat double timed with excitement and panic. Now I just had to kill time before he arrived and we started our epic New Year's first date.

I went to the Friday evening farmer's market across the street and ran into my Brooklyn friend Dani, who was working at the nut booth. He was wearing a maroon velvet mini skirt and go-go boots. I was turned on by his courage to wear femme clothes even to the farmer's market. I felt myself being abducted by his hazel teddy bear eyes, but I reminded myself that he was in a monogamous relationship with psychedelics.

He sampled me local pecans and pistachios. Then he took me on a locals-only tour of the market, teaching me about new varieties of citrus. We tried sour little kumquats, you can eat the skin. I had my first persimmon, whose flavor, we agreed, was umami—the illusive sixth taste. The abundance of food and the carnival glow of the hanging lights got me into a festive mood. But as soon as I said goodbye, the uncertainty returned.

It was 8pm. Still a few hours before the ball dropped but my heart was already sunk. I was in mourning. Death is as painful for a hope, a plan, or an illusion. Where was he?

I stopped in at Walgreens and sampled a matte grey nail polish on each of my nails. Usually I would have bought it out of respect, but I was feeling reckless. Nothing seemed certain now. Not tonight, not tomorrow, never. Pablo not texting dis-qualified all we'd shared. It wasn't just him, either. Maybe all my beliefs and hopes in life were just illusions to avoid the true chaos. I looked at myself in a distorted foil mirror next to the lipsticks. Why couldn't I find love? What was wrong with me that made me undesirable? Why couldn't I see it? Emotion erupted in my bloodstream. I hated him for ignoring me but also hated myself for not being good enough for him. I wanted to destroy something. I had to leave and walk it off before I demolished the cosmetic section. I rushed out the sliding doors holding my wet nails out so not to smudge them. Then someone texted. I carefully reached into my bag for my phone, but still messed up my nails. It wasn't him.

Under an orange tree blinking with Christmas lights, I called an Uber. The fruit looked fake. I pulled one off to check and it was real! This was Christmas in LA, citrus instead of snow. When I got to my friends' house I smelled the campfire smoke. The dark stairs up the side of the hill they lived on were covered in dried bougainvillea flowers. It looked poetic, the un-swept potpourri of L.A. In the yard people were bundled up in the coats and sweaters they only got to wear a few weeks of the year. I was still feeling shook up and went to sit on the couch by the fire. They had brought the couch outside to clear the living room for dancing. I could see out to the mountains of Pasadena, and the city lights pulsed like embers. They had thrown bougainvillea flowers into the fire as kindling. I sat on the couch and watched the pink paper lanterns lift up as they caught fire. I wanted the fire to transform how I was feeling. I poured my emotions onto the flames like psychic lighter fluid. I recalled what Dana once said: "You give your personal power away when you wait for someone else to validate you. No one can give you what you haven't yet given to yourself." The fire blazed up.

"How ya doin' buddy?" The words snapped me out of my introspection. It was my friend Ruby. "An elixir for your heart, young Skywalker." He offered me a white ceramic cup, "coconut milk chai with mushrooms. Just enough for vibeys."

I'd met Ruby at the Body Actualized Center in Brooklyn.

He's a musician, DJ, and a raw food wizard. He has a sharp mind, a big heart, and copper red hair. We sipped the chai by the fire, then he took my hand and led me to the dance floor.

Sage smoke filled the room like fog. It glowed blue from a clip light in the corner. The music was groovy '80s electro soul. It was a portal out of Earth's pain. My body was getting tingly. The blue sage clouds felt like we were dancing in the sky. The room was going somewhere, through space, traveling away from yesterday, from the past, towards a new year, a new vibe. A sad thought would distract me—did I do something wrong with Pablo to make him not want to hang out? But then I'd be snapped out of it from the other people around me dancing, amping me up with their energy. One girl in particular, who had a sideways ponytail and a lavender metallic biker jacket. My emotions became fuel for kinetic dance moves.

Ruby put on the '90s rave song "It's a Fine Day." It was a reassuring message as we headed into the month when Trump would be inaugurated. But we would dance and create our own bubbles of freaky freedom no matter what. The music paused in a shimmery breakdown like a shooting star and everyone moved like seaweed. Then the beat dropped again and the room jumped on it. Squatting and bouncing, back to animals, back to sperm bouncing towards eggs, spaceships crash landing on Earth. Dancing moves matter back to the energy all things come from.

I felt my spirit rebuilding itself. Like in bodybuilding where you tear your muscles so they grow back bigger, guys kept tearing my heart to swell it bigger with inner Love. It felt triumphant to have fun even without a New Year's kiss. My friends, the mushrooms and the music had held me, and brought me back to myself.

2

Leaving Woodstock

I arrived to the Woodstock festival 47 years late. Luckily, the town keeps the vibe alive. I had moved there to connect to Nature after eight years in the city, and join my fellow hippie freaks. "PEACE" is written everywhere. Tourists visit, as do weekenders from NYC. You can get anything in tie dye. The town retains the politics and playfulness of the hippie movement. Wizard beards are common. No one cares if bells jangle from your pants hem. I wanted to find the equivalent of the hippie movement of today and live a different way.

But winter in my cabin was isolating. Everything was dormant, both Nature and people. Every day I drove down to town for a dose of human interaction at The Lonely Loaf Cafe. The staff were my only social outlet. They felt like family and I tipped them as such.

I got to know one of the cafe regulars, Allen, who could always be found at the window stools. He was a local celebrity, known for being part of The Factory and acting in Bertolucci films. He taught me bohemian history while we sipped to-go cups. During the Summer of Love, he lived in Los Angeles.

"Things were so free back then. You would have loved it. LA was smaller and you never knew where you were going to end up. They had this really strong acid called Orange Sunshine."

His bony hands were like polished wood knots, his eyes like crystal balls. I bought us another round of almond croissants and he bit in with the good side of his teeth, avoiding the missing ones.

"You should have known Cameron. She was a real witch artist. Her paintings were alive. Someone tried to buy one and she told them 'you can't handle this painting' and didn't sell it. And you know her husband was the first rocket man."

Outside the window, hippie ancestors maneuvered the grey slush in boots and scarves. In 1969, they were my age. I spiraled off thinking about the mystery and mercilessness of time. I loved imagining the spirit of the 1960s but I wanted to find the Woodstock of now. Was I ready to retire in this small town or did I have more adventures in me? Allen's stories of LA had planted a seed.

I frequented Woodstock's metaphysical bookstore Mirabai. It was on the first floor of a Victorian house. The shop was bright and clean, like a classroom, and smelled of decades of incense. I befriended the owner Audrey who wore Renaissance fair skirts and had a beaming smile. She introduced me to the "Ascended Masters" section, which was tucked away be-hind Self Help. The shelf where things got weird.

"This is the shelf for dreamers. I think you're just the type for it," she said with a wink. These were the books that taught how to activate your DNA. The book covers looked like sci-fi spirituality. One had a huge egg hatching in the forest, with Earth and a starry night inside. Skimming it, I gathered it was channeled from aliens. "Be careful what you think," they warned, "because it becomes reality." Damn it, enough already! I waas tired of hearing the same manifestation talk but it didn't work for me. I wanted to pitch the book across the shop to knock the tarot decks over like bowling pins. But instead I calmly slid the book back into its place in the alpha-betical order of things.

Were you just supposed to ignore and starve the negative thoughts and feelings until they withered away? I'd been try-ing that for years and they still came back, like weeds, worse. They seemed to just get stronger. While I loved the cover art, the philosophy of New Age Ascension wasn't working for me—there was no guidance on how to deal with gritty feel-ings. What about trauma? History? What about social ine-quality? I kept looking for that book that would help me learn how to access Divinity while still remaining part of society.

On my way out I glimpsed the back cover of *The Venus Juice Cookbook*; a veiled woman carried a white cake decorated with flowers. I opened it and drank in colorful pages of splattered juices, chia pudding, and long, flowing hair.

"Oh that just came in, isn't it fabulous?" Audrey said from behind the counter, her eyes twinkling behind Mrs. Claus glasses.

I rarely bought books from Mirabai, just sort of browsed them like a bumble bee pollinating flower-to-flower. But this was worth my $30. Money was tight since I'd quit managing the events at Maha Rose in Brooklyn. I still went to the city to lead breathwork workshops and private sessions, but I was mostly living on credit. Now that I was 30, I didn't want to ask my family for money anymore. I knew my financial insecurity stressed them out. I charged the cookbook. Audrey handed it to me in a flat paper bag and then we exchanged namastes.

Over the next week my cabin transformed into a Venus Juice oasis. I soaked cashews and blended them with water to make nut milk. I went to the health food store for raw cacao, coconut oil and seaweed. I was under the tutelage of beautiful Briana Lemaire Taylor, the book's author, who had learned how to be healthy and spiritual, and ran a boutique juice shop in Los Angeles. The book quenched something deep. Briana had done what I wanted to do: to be successful by expressing yourself, creating something that helps people be more healthy and happy. And she showed you could do it in style. I felt thirsty for life as I looked at the photos of her Frank Gehry house, her quirky still lifes and food altars. She shined with a radiant beauty and stress-free vitality I could feel.

I couldn't wait to milk all types of nuts. Brazil, almond, cashew—anything that was over $10 a pound seemed suitable. I'd originally heard of Briana on a viral video of someone reading her daily menu and itemizing the cost of the ingredients. It was funny how expensive it all was, but I was finding it was true—I spent $43 on three ingredients for her chocolate recipe. I charged the superfoods and went back up the icy hill to my house to make raw cacao dipped apricots.

Many signs from the Universe were pointing me towards California. And now Venus Juice was too. A snowstorm trapped me in the cabin. I had cancelled plowing to save money. That week I went deep into the cookbook. I began to wonder: maybe my emotional problems were from gluten? Sugar? Dairy? Cut them all out and my life would be as gorgeous as Brianna's. I listened to California rock as I ate chia pudding. The sunny photos of cacti in the book made me wonder if my problem was that I was just in the wrong place. Was I meant to be in LA? Brianna made it look so gorgeous. Maybe my soul just needed a beach? I wanted to live the Venus Juice way. Brianna had tapped into a neo-hippie aesthetic, and made an easeful state of being into a luxury product. This seemed like success to me; to be able to transform who you are into a sellable product. She was a hippie entrepreneur. Maybe I could be, too.

As I was finishing the apricots, the gas company called: my payment had failed. I licked raw chocolate from my fingers as I listened. The extra heat had come to $1000, it maxed out my credit card. I gave them another card number. Living upstate and barely working in the city wasn't working. In the last of my life coaching sessions, Dana encouraged me to see my value and bring my spirit into form. I repeated the mantras we made every day and saw myself stirring a cauldron of silver mercury. But I couldn't land on a more realistic symbol for my work—what would I do with the liquid silver? It was my potential without a firm shape ... I was too blocked to actually believe in my own self, and my work as a healer. Worse, I had trouble fully trusting my intuition, my gut, a requirement if I wanted to excel in the field. In art, I doubted myself too, never thinking anything I made was good enough. It seemed hopeless.

That night, sitting at the kitchen table lost in my phone screen, I saw my friend Meg was subletting her apartment in East LA for April. That would give me a month's notice to break my lease and pack up the cabin. April also happened to be when Pablo, the Painter from Portland, would be in L.A. doing a residency. We had quit talking after he stood me up on New Year's, but the loneliness of the cabin had made me reach out to begin our virtual romance again. Maybe it could still happen? I put on Harry Nillson's twangy "Everybody's Talking" because the words came into my head: "I'm going where the Sun keeps shining, through the pouring rain, where the weather suits my clothes."

The prospect of the move excited me. Maybe this was the place I'd finally find my people. When I first learned about Indigo Children—a new generation born with spiritual consciousness—it confirmed why I'd always felt so weird. I identified myself as an Indigo Child immediately. Indigos are here to evolve the planet, but also find it hard to fit in with our current systems. We're the dreamers and the revolutionaries. The idea was comforting and relieved me from feeling like such misfit. But where were all the other Indigo people? Indigos come into the world sensitive, intuitive, gentle and compassionate. But with this, a lot of baggage develops if they have to guard that openness. Some Indigos turn to addiction to distract and numb. In my case, I overdeveloped my intellect to try to make sense of it all. Maybe I could finally live from my heart in LA.

In the final days of my time in the cabin upstate, I got really sick. I had made a tincture from Reishi mushrooms a friend and I had foraged while hiking. I wanted to complete the process of making the tincture before I left and not waste the sacred mushrooms. Reishi was revered in ancient China as a longevity tonic, bestowing peace of spirit and boosting the immune system. I had researched making a Reishi tincture online. It was a two-step process: soak them in vodka, then strain them, boil the mushrooms in water, and then blend the vodka with an equal amount of the mushroom tea. It was while the mushrooms boiled that I started to worry: what if they weren't actually Reishi? I recognized the waxy brown ears from herb shops in Chinatown. When we spotted them on the side of a tree my friend and I were psyched and agreed they were definitely Reishi. But I wished I had gotten a second opinion.

In my secluded cabin studies I had taken herbalist Asia Suler's online class "Reishi: Key to the Otherworld." She said the mushroom was a portal opener. Not psychedelic, but something that awakens the intuition, soothes the heart, and aligns us to the spiritual side of life. I was about to go through a portal with my move to L.A., so maybe it was the moment to imbibe? Studying herbs was one way to learn to listen to Nature's rhythm and intelligence. Nature is trying to help us. I started to feel sad about leaving the creeks and moss-covered fairy land. The rich world beyond matter was palpable in these magical forests. I remembered the glimpses I'd had in Nature of being okay, of being in harmony with something greater. Fairy forests don't pay the bills, though.

I ladled the Reishi tea into my *Beauty and the Beast* mug. The alcohol had boiled off. It had a bitter cardboard taste. I wanted to feel proud of my foraging and wizardry, but instead, I felt an avalanche of dread that I had just poisoned myself. I looked again on the mushroom identification site and re-read the recipe. I'd done it all correctly, but I didn't trust myself.

Later, I would see this habit of mine was the source of all my problems. It wasn't that I was doing life wrong; it was that I was constantly doubting myself. My phone dinged with a new Tinder message from a long-haired dancer I was planning to go on a date with in the city before I left. Life always brings new hope.

Then my stomach shifted into reverse. I ran to the bathroom and released the tea along with all the expensive raw food I'd had that day. At least my body was working: it sensed something off in the biome and was doing its job to rebalance. After the eruption was over, I laid wilted on the couch until I was summoned back to the toilet. There's how you imagine things to be and then how they actually turn out. I wanted my life to be graceful and beautiful, like the cookbook, but it also has its sick, gross and sad moments. Most disappointing was that I'd have to cancel the Tinder date. With the handicap of the Reishi volcano clearing out my system, I would need every last minute to pack up and move out of the cabin. I tapped out a message, but was too weak to fix the typos. It was cryptic: "Too sock sorta I can't hang before I leave."

I felt the grip in my stomach again and rushed back to the bathroom. There was still so much to pack. I wanted to return the blue glass goblets to the Free Tibet thrift store, back to their source, so they could be found by someone else. And my stomach felt like it was doing the same thing; releasing all it had gotten from Woodstock, emptying back to the source. I'd rest for 15 minutes, and then pack until my stomach started to hurt again.

The night I took my last load to the storage unit on Route 28, I felt destiny like a magnet, my moves flowing in a current beyond my control, blown on by a cosmic breeze. I didn't know if or when I would be back. It was pouring but not too cold. My headlights lit up the rain. The silhouettes of pine trees were all around. I'd given up staying dry and splashed in the puddle around my car as I loaded boxes in. My stomach ached from the diarrhea and not having eaten for two days. After I shut the storage door and locked it with a padlock, I felt the gravity my ancestors must have felt when they left for America from Eastern Europe. There's always a gamble when you leave something behind for what you hope will be better. I was doing this so my children would never have to get snowed in. So they could eat spirulina ice cream in the most innovative health food stores. My corduroy jacket was soaked; but I knew it would dry right up in the L.A. sunshine.

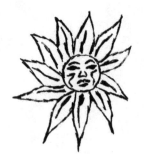

3
Arrival in LA

When I got to Adriana's from the airport the Sun was rising. She let me stay with her until my sublet started. From her window, the palm trees and thousands of houses on the hills started coming to light. The joy I felt as the orange glow filled the room made me grab the guitar off the wall. I played "Strong Enough to Be My Man" by Sheryl Crow. Adriana sang along from bed. I felt energized and inspired by LA, but my body was singing a different tune. I was still under the influence of whatever microbes, mycelium, or nerves were in my gut.

I waited until the walk-in doctor's office opened and then drove to Pasadena. She had grey spiky hair and wore green rectangular glasses. I told her about moving out of my cabin and the homemade Reishi tincture. "Sounds like you've been under a lot of stress, it might just be that," she said. This was disappointing, as the idea of dying from mushroom poisoning had grown on me over the past few days. It seemed like a good enough place to finish my story. I'd chased my dreams, but had gotten my mushrooms wrong.

I'm not afraid to die. I imagine the afterlife is a realm of Love and ethereal minimalism. Whatever happens when we die, we will all get to experience it. I was ready for the news as the doctor typed in silence. I was relieved that I wouldn't have to figure my life out if the Reishi won. But the doctor re-routed my exit strategy. "I think it will pass. Do the BRAT diet—bananas, rice, applesauce, toast—and I'll have you do a stool sample." I left feeling renewed and grateful.

After I dropped off my stool sample to the Davita testing center, I went to the Starbucks across the street. The familiar flavors are a comfort food that bring me back to high school. I got an iced chai. The banana bread looked good in the case—that would fulfill both banana and toast on the BRAT diet—so I got one. The familiarity of the cool, sweet milk with the greasy bread calmed me. My stomach settled for the first time in days. I wished I could find the chai feeling within myself. I couldn't rely on Starbucks for something stable and consistent to hold on to. Sitting on the patio next to a fountain, watching cars enter the freeway, I felt the good side of uncertainty—anything could happen. When I relaxed into the free-fall, I felt the exhilaration of freedom I'd been craving. I grabbed my guitar from the car and strummed Sheryl Crow to the honking cars entering the 110 Freeway. When you first arrive in a new place your senses and imagination are re-awakened.

I drove back to Echo Park to walk around. I saw the Latino and Filipino history of the area in the fading murals and old businesses. Eventually, I made it to The House of Intuition, which sits precariously close to the edge of a cliff above Sunset. It looks like it landed there after a tornado, squishing a witch, leaving her feet dangling out. The black house has the word INTUITION painted on it in huge letters, as a billboard to passing traffic. On the street, a sign says "Your Intuition Led You Here" by the stairwell up to the house. Each step was painted with an astrological glyph. I couldn't resist walking up, planet by planet.

Half-way up the stairs was a landing with white gravel and pine bushes. A guy was meditating on the bench. It was too good to be true. Was this an apparition? He was wearing a sequined jacket with no shirt on underneath. He sat so still, he seemed to have switched into a photosynthesis state. I didn't want to disturb his meditation. I kept walking up the stairs but I felt drawn back to sit with him. Meditating looked so good right now. Beyond his tan and body, this guy emanated a golden peace. I quietly sat down on the other bench.

I closed my eyes and heard traffic echo down from Sunset. I smelled the incense from the psychics above. The living room has been converted into a crystal shop with the bedrooms reserved for tarot readings and mediums. I opened my eyes to look at the guy's jacket shimmering again. Could I have both the outer glitter and the inner glitter? I closed my eyes again. It's easier to enter meditation when someone else is anchoring it. I listened to traffic to try to dis-engage from my mind. The shaking struts of a big truck; do I want to move here? Maybe I could work at The House of Intuition? A honk brought me back to mindfulness. Maybe I could become a famous guru? But how could I be a guru when I could barely meditate myself? I thought I'd quit and go up to the shop. Shopping is more satisfying than witnessing your own neuroses. I peeked and he was still there, motionless as a statue, so I decided to stay. As you resist the urge to get up, to get anywhere, your energy settles and you feel the layer of yourself beyond the chatter. I've learned to sit past the point when I can't stand it anymore, because that's how you get out beyond your own resistance.

I hadn't landed and paused in weeks. I felt us sitting together in the topaz sunshine. So much is happening beyond our control. I let out a sigh. The traffic sounds died down, birds were chirping. I hadn't felt peace in a while and sponged it in.

"Hey! Luke!"

I blinked awake to see him smiling.

"How you been buddy?!"

I still couldn't tell if he was a human or an Angelic apparition. He could sense from my delayed response that I didn't recognize him.

"It's me Oz, from Body Actualized"

"Wow hey! Thanks for the meditation."

He used to come to my yoga classes. He was normal back then—a jeans and a t-shirt guy. Now he was an enlightened freak.

"You look so different, I didn't recognize you."

"Ya LA changes you."

"And you're so tan. I'm jealous."

"Ya, I do yoga outside every day. I wish there was a place like Body here."

"I miss it too." We paused back into the peace of meditation for a moment.

I'd met him when he had just moved from the Midwest to Brooklyn. Body Actualized was a community space with yoga classes by day, and a speakeasy club by night. People were waking up and exploring consciousness, both through spirituality and psychedelics. The moment had passed once the rent went up, and forced the characters from that scene to figure how to live in the real world. I had heard through a friend that Oz was homeless in LA, but he made it look pretty good.

"So, what have you been up to?" I asked.

"I've been DJing around. But I lost my phone, so now I can't anymore. My jacket got stolen last night with my phone and wallet in it."

"Damn. That sucks."

"Ya, I've been staying with this girl but I haven't been able to get a hold of her since I lost it. I was supposed to DJ her art opening and get paid $200."

"It's cool you're DJing," I said, remembering when he was just a sprout to the nightlife.

The peace from the meditation dissipated as I realized the situation he was in. I'd seen his incomprehensible Facebook posts. He used to work at a restaurant but I doubt he could hold down a job now. Would he even want to? His path was romantic but scary to me. We were both starting to sweat from the Sun and his aroma ripened: socks marinated in sweat. I wanted to help him, but I couldn't have him dependent on me.

"I should get going," I said.

"Alright, well I'm always around here so I'll see you."

I walked down the stairs and kept walking on Sunset.

How to be as free as possible, while also existing within the money system? And still showering? What if you reach for your dreams, leap, and the net doesn't appear? To have any amount of comfort you have to stay in the system. Either give all your juice to your day job, or figure out how to make money off your passion. There was no place in the world for artists and mystics unless they worked out how to profit off of it. Los Angeles was home to rich artists, actors, and musicians. To make art and get rich from it, that would be living the dream.

I reached the spinning Happy Foot/Sad Foot sign at a podiatrists office. It looked like a prop from Pee Wee's Playhouse.

I wanted to always be happy, but I wondered if the spinning happy/sad dynamic wasn't maybe the nature of Earth? As the sign spun, I thought about Karma and who gets what situations in life; is it just chance? Some people are homeless, while others get famous. I walked away, my happy foot leading my sad foot.

It was around noon and I passed a parking lot with all the windshields blazing like fireworks, reflecting the Sun. Then I saw the sign for Venus Juice. The orb logo brought a near divine devotion in my heart. I'd made it! As I walked in the door I was bathed in the soft light of a frosted skylight. I got goosebumps, from both air conditioning and from the excitement.

Entering the shop feels like boarding a spaceship. It is ethereal, and minimal. The potted plants and rocks on the groung look like a Japanese garden. "Welcome, what brings you in today?" the pink haired woman behind the counter asked me.

"Hi, just browsing and looking for a juice."

"Well you came to the right place. Let me sample you something." She opened the refrigerator and pulled out a few bottles.

"So I'm going to have you start with blue, then red, then green," she said as she poured them into little plastic cups.

They tasted like organic gourmet Gatorade. I went with the boldest one: ginger, kale, parsley, lemon and celery.

"Great, would you like to add any herbs?" She handed me

the menu of supplements. I looked and saw Reishi, which I would be avoiding until I heard back from the doctor. "Oh, I'll try Mucuna, the happiness booster."

"Okay, I think a banana will really help bring the flavors together, the Mucuna is bitter, and I will make it a nice, thick smoothie for you."

"Yum, that sounds great."

Plus, it would get me another banana on my BRAT diet! I browsed the raw crackers. At $7 a pack they were a splurge, but it seemed pretty close to toast, fulfilling another T, so I went for it.

"Here you are! Try it and let me know what you think." She placed the swampy green smoothie on the counter.

It was cold and sweet with a minty, fish food aftertaste. It tasted like my homeless friend smelled. My brain froze in a moment of enlightenment, inundated by minerals and vitamins.

"It's amazing, thank you!"

"So altogether it's $29."

Shocked, I swallowed wrong and coughed. I smiled and pulled out my wallet. How was I going to afford my new LA lifestyle?

I finished my smoothie on the bench in front of the shop. I read the bottle: "Mineralizer. Immune Support. Cleansing." I could feel it working. People wonder whether stuff like this is placebo. But isn't buying anything placebo? Having a fancy car doesn't do anything for you besides make you think you are special. Luxury is all imagination: "Buying this will make your life better." But people don't demand proof or measurements of how luxury works the way they do herbs. I wished people were as skeptical of all the stuff we buy as they are about wellness and spirituality. I felt like a wilted plant perking back up. This was more than just the hydration; it was the idea, the look, the feeling of the juice, too, that lifted me up. I would be happy just drinking juice in the Sun. I imagined sitting in front of the shop with a cardboard sign that said, "Need money for juice."

Next I walked to Plato, the Australian skincare shop, to see if my friend Ruby was working. Ruby had transformed his charisma into a steady income and was one of the better adapted people to come out of the Body Actualized community since it closed. The door was propped open and I could feel the air conditioning coaxing me into the clean, rosemary world inside.

"Can I help you find anything today?" the clerk with oversized circular glasses asked me.

"Is Ruby here?"

"Oh yes, Rubin, let me fetch him."

He came out like a character on a sitcom, entering to canned applause. "There he is," we said at the same time. Ruby made two guns with his hands as he came in for a hug.

He was living in an '80s comedy and I loved having a cameo. We hugged for a long time. It wasn't until a customer came in that we snapped back to reality. Ruby let me go and brushed off his apron and welcomed the customer to the shop. A man in a tank top and flip flops with a cocker spaniel on a leash.

I browsed the shelves while Ruby worked his magic. He washed the guy's hands with $40 hand soap, exfoliated them and patted them dry with a towel. "This is our after-sun toner, very important here in the desert." He misted the orbit of the man's head obsequiously. "I'll take all of it," the guy said. The cocker spaniel, as obedient as his owner, let out a sigh from the floor.

"Baby, you're getting burned be careful!" Ruby said, and misted around me with the after-sun toner. Whether it was the ginger smoothie at Venus Juice or just my body healing, my hunger was back and I hadn't eaten in days. "When's your break? Wanna go get tacos?" I asked him.

"It's Taco Tuesday. Did you know? The fish tacos are only $2.50!" Ruby said. He checked with his co-worker and came back with sunglasses on and his apron off and we walked to the outdoor taco restaurant.

I ordered a side of beans and rice, getting me an R for my BRAT. All I needed now was applesauce. We sat at the metal table waiting for our order. "Number 34" a crackly intercom announced. I went up to grab my tray.

"Do you want salsa?" I saw the plastic containers stacked and the texture was the same as applesauce. It would do the trick, I figured, as a substitute.

"Yes, thank you." The universe provides, but in unexpected ways.

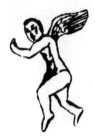

4

The Painter from Portland

Pablo and I had picked up talking again after he'd stood me up New Year's. We both missed the buzz of flirting. When my sublet started I sat at the kitchen table all day thinking, writing, waiting. Now we were both in LA, it was frustrating because he would always respond, "I can't I'm painting," if he even responded at all when I invited him to hang out.

I wish I was as focused and dedicated to my work as he was. I tried to use the time to plan my workshop but instead I re-watched the video of him jacking off with Electric Light Orchestra playing in the background. It cracked me up because it was such a goofy band to masturbate to. But that's why I loved Pablo, because he was smart and had offbeat humor. It is rare to meet someone who is dialed to your same radio signal of weird. Your freakquency. That first week in LA I just sat at home. I felt boxed in again, waiting for Pablo to text, when I thought LA would be this big new adventure. I felt like I was swinging from a trapeze waiting for him to reach out and grab on.

I was preparing for the breathwork workshop I was teaching at Yogala in Echo Park on Easter. In my healer training with Mike Kelly he emphasized Self-Love. When you are loving you, your actions spiral from your heart and connect you to grace. When you act from lack of Self-Love, you reach out desperately for something to fill you; this is where people get desperate, addicted, abusive and eventually sick. That is the low vibe energy. I was trying to map it out in my notebook, because I want to understand things in my own words and experiences, not just repeat spiritual jargon. High vibe is when you feel joyful, light, clear. It is why I had come to LA. I hoped LA was the right climate for me to figure out how to live in the high vibes.

I filled the days walking around Highland Park. I saw Deb's Park on the map and walked there on a frontage road, separated from the freeway by a chain-link fence. Passing homeless encampments, I came to a worn footpath and started up the mountain that has a great view of downtown. I was the only one around and I made up a song and sang it out loud: "peace and Love to myself, shine it out to everyone else, high vibe, high vibe I choose my vibe." At the top there was a swing hanging from a tree branch. I pumped until I was going fast enough to jump off and be airborne for a second, and crash, like I always did on the playground.

I remembered how I'd run away from home when I was

four and walked to my aunt Bee's house. I had packed my pre-school backpack with a snake identification book, my Malibu Barbie, and two cans of Coke for me and Bee to share once I got there. Bee was one of the only people I felt safe sharing my dolls with. Her house was decorated in pastel colors and we would blast UB40 and Sade tapes. But she wasn't home when 4-year-old me arrived that day, and the neighbors called the cops to find my parents. This memory connected me to a great part of myself, my bravery and boldness. But it was also one of my wounds, that constant searching and feeling alone.

My life coach Dana had explained that I had to value the bedrock layer of who I was. Not because I did everything right, but because I had the right to exist. As I hiked back, I felt strong, healthy, and happy to just be alive. When I had told her about coming to LA for the month, and seeing Pablo the Painter, she said "you have to find your healthy middle. Reach out and let them meet you halfway. You can't receive what you can't give yourself first." I was trying to photo-synthesize the feeling of deep fulfillment and sexy joy as I walked home, nearly getting hit by a car exiting the 110 freeway too fast.

That evening I watched the sunset out the window. The palm trees against the orange sky were more poignant in person. I had heard LA was just desert before it was landscaped into an oasis by real estate developers. The palm trees were brought here to brand the city as a paradise. Even if they were imported, I loved what they stood for: dreams, migration, new possibilities, glamour, creativity. LA was almost cooler because it was such a vision. The same way NYC is an industrial miracle, LA is a sprawling garden automobile emerald city. In both art and city development a vision is brought into reality. The interplay between the imagination and how it takes shape in the physical world fascinates me. Was it hard work, luck, manifestation, or a combination of all three? I recited my affirmation, "my life is fabulously fulfilling," and saw myself driving with a boyfriend through a sunny canyon. I hoped it would work, that Pablo would like me. An astrologer once told me about my square aspect of Venus and Neptune: "you'll learn." Learn what? From my studies I gathered it had to do with illusions or dreams around Love and partnership.

When the palm trees looked like cut paper silhouettes, Pablo finally texted:

"Wanna come over to the studio and let me cast your foot for a sculpture? I just got a handle of vodka."

I've always wanted to be someone's muse, so was happy to share my foot. I don't really drink, but could let it slide. "I'm down" I replied, and started getting ready. I showered and then combed my shiny hair in the mirror. I realized my ability to make myself hot was an attempt to be desired. There's a beauty that comes from self-love, clipping your nails and filing them gently, honoring and caring for your vessel. But there's another step where you add on and modify yourself in worry that you won't be enough as you are. You turn yourself into someone's Ken or Barbie doll in hopes of seducing them. So many gay guys work so hard to be accepted in a certain image, to be desired. I wish we could be more caring knowing we've all experienced alienation and bigotry growing up.

As I put on a black mesh t-shirt and sprayed myself with patchouli perfume, he sent another text: "There are some friends over, too, that cool?"

Confusion, anger and disappointment erupted inside me. I pulled my arm back to throw my phone out the window, but I knew I'd have to pay for it to be fixed. I wilted onto the bed. I thought this was a date? I hadn't imagined our first hang to involve other people. I wanted him to myself, not hang in a crowd. A single sentence activated every pain and fear in me. "There are some friends over, too, that cool?" killed something I had been hoping for. The dream I had of him, of us, of the sacredness of our internet plans coming to life after nine months.

I drafted and deleted responses: "Hey ... I thought it was going to be just us" ... no, too sentimental. I hoped he wasn't watching the pulsing ellipsis that showed my deliberation. "I want you alone"... no, too desperate. I finally texted him, "Never mind, not tonight." I sat in the charged silence. I wanted to cry but was too pissed off. I didn't know what else to do, so I went on a walk.

Everything changes in the dark. The colors of the flowers disappear. Sub-tropical LA turns eerie. Hidden things return. Every dog bark and rustle in the leaves scared me. This is the pitfall of having a sensitive nervous system: you are insightful, emotional, even psychic, but also skittish. In Brooklyn, I would have walked over the bridge and gone to a late-night bookshop. In LA, the only thing I knew would be open was the taco truck, so I headed there. I tried to practice what I preached and choose high vibes rather than spin into feeling rejected and betrayed. I power walked down Figueroa Ave, huffing as I went faster and harder. Moving the Energy, I remembered, was part of my lesson plan. But how was I supposed to be a healing teacher when I was so fucked up?

My anger came to a rolling boil. I broke into a run, wind coming in my black mesh shirt. I flailed my arms and shook my head trying to shake the feelings out as I jogged. Someone honked their horn and I froze. I had to love myself, I remembered. I could disrupt this pattern with new energy. I felt lucid. The store signs across the street glowed. What did I love about myself? I love myself for being so emotional and dramatic. I laughed, but it was true. The traffic lights turned green. I took a deep breath and walked towards the blinking taco truck. I had a newfound compassion for the chunk of roasting meat. I know how you feel, I psychically communicated to it. We are all being gradually roasted and softened.

I ordered an horchata. The sweet rice and cinnamon calmed me back to peace. The night was cool and light. As I walked home I thought: maybe I'd share this experience at my workshop. Mike Kelly said, "don't wait until you are healed to help others." Maybe being honest with what I was dealing with, and how I was getting through, would help people more than appearing to be perfect and have it all together?

On April 14th, the night of his opening, Pablo texted: "Are you still coming tonight? Sorry I've been MIA. Been super busy putting the show together."

I typed "Maybe," deleted it. Retyped "maybe," and sent it.

None of my friends could accompany me, but I'd come all the way to LA for him—I had to go to the opening. I felt both excited and anxious. I used the tingly energy to compose the most extreme outfit possible, given the limited options in my suitcase. I went with shorts overalls, mesh t-shirt, gold socks, lace-up platform sandals, and my black velvet cap. I looked like a character from the '90s TV show Blossom, but with a beard and bleached hair.

The gallery was in a warehouse in Mid-City. I walked up the wooden staircase feeling effervescent and woozy. I'd been too anxious to eat dinner. The room was full of wood squares that made floating walls for the paintings. The crowd mingled among the paintings, creating a lively chatter. I felt shy not knowing anyone there and grabbed a beer just to have something to hold and do. Sipping, I started looking at the paintings. It was both mythic and grunge. The best piece was an oil painting of a nude guy looking at his distorted reflection in swirling water. I wanted to be the one he painted. The ability to create worlds is sexy to me. And this was a world I wanted to live in. He captured the beauty of being lost in the Universe.

There was completeness to the paintings even without a point or a reason. A fork twisted with spaghetti in front of foliage. The images were naive but also fresh. They made me feel ok to not know the point or destination of my life, that everything is weirdly beautiful without a reason. He'd made clay hand mirrors, with tin foil as the blunt, incoherent reflections. The show cast a spell by seeing ancient things in new ways.

He emerged from behind one of the paintings. We had a moment of recognizing each other for the first time in real life. He was different—skinnier, had cut his hair short. But I quickly connected the photos to the reality. He smiled and reached for a hug. "Hey, I'm so glad you came." I felt the crook of his low back for a few extra seconds, amazed to finally touch him.

"This is amazing, I'm so impressed," I said.

He smiled. "Thanks. It means a lot you came." There was a beat of silence. I smiled at him, feeling the suspense of reaching out and hoping he'd reach back on the trapeze. Someone grabbed his shoulder and started introducing him, "This is the artist ..." "Sorry, gotta go" he waved. I went back to sipping my beer. Alone. Just another show goer. Not a muse, a special guest, or a lover. I thought he'd whisk me to a closet or alley, and we'd come back 6 minutes later, after a kiss that had felt like infinity. There's how you think Love will be, and how it actually turns out.

I was saved from being alone by my outfit. Fashion is always a conversation starter. I was talking about overalls to some guys when Pablo re-emerged and introduced me, "This is Luke, he's from Brooklyn"

"Where do you guys know each other from?" one of the guys asked. We looked at each other. "Uh, instagram?" I said. The guys nodded in chill approval and took sips from their beers. Then someone else grabbed Pablo, "I want to introduce you to the curator from ...". He held his glass up in cheers and went to attend to his duties as man of the hour. I hung around, met some LA queers, but it didn't seem like Pablo was going to be able to connect, or even wanted to. I left without saying bye.

Waking up the next day I had a similar sense of non-belief I had felt the morning after Trump got elected. But this was much more personal. It wouldn't affect the whole world, the way Trump did, but still weighed as heavily. A bubble had popped, something dark began now in its aftermath: reality. Were all my dreams illusions that would end in rude awakenings?

Adriana came over and I felt blessed by all her mantra tattoos as we hugged. She French-braided my hair while I told her the story. She had just been written up in the *New York Times* as the healing hair witch who blended her cuts with her intuitive advice and guidance. "Fuck these un-requited guys. You need someone who can appreciate and honor you! Rejection is protection."

When Adriana left, the silence and pain returned. I felt weak and laid in bed. It was weird to feel bad on such a bright spring day. I didn't think it was possible to feel this dark in LA. I thought the Sun dried out sadness. I knew if I did breathwork, it would move the haze and heaviness in my body. But I was too tired to focus. breathwork works by moving the life force carried in our breathing, which stimulates our subtle energy body. It gets stagnant energy unstuck. Seeing how important moving was for me when I felt stuck, exercise and walking were becoming a part of my healing tool kit. I plopped by the shoe rack and slowly laced my platform sandals to walk.

The aimless walking got me feeling my body again. I passed a donut shop and strip club. When I feel embodied, I am less distracted by thought and intuitive downloads come through. The understanding streamed in, from the Sun, from my heart: my pain and sadness were from my own expectations. I had to face my inner lack of Love that had become so needy and fixated on getting it from somebody. I paused to pet a flowering mimosa tree in the Chase bank parking lot. These guys I'd fallen for were all artists. I had secretly hoped that if someone powerful loved me, then I'd feel validated to express myself under the umbrella of their Love. I had to become my own artist, love my own spark. A few tears streamed, a release.

The moment that compassion in my heart arrived, I saw a hardware store across the street and had an intuitive flash: I needed a chain necklace. This experience was making me go goth. I walked into the shop and bought a foot of silver chain and a padlock. I put it around my neck and locked myself up. It was an instant symbol for the wholeness, strength and boundaries I needed. I wasn't going to give myself away anymore hoping to get the validation and Love I needed to give myself. Self-love is badass, I realized from the weight of the chain on my neck.

At its best, fashion communicates emotions. My new necklace said: Fragile, don't touch. And, FUCK YOU. The chain would remind me of my new direction every time I'd see it. It was a symbol of me taking back my power. No more waiting for texts back, when I could be focused on loving myself harder, so I didn't find myself in these painful situations anymore.

As I walked on York Avenue, I posted a selfie wearing the chain necklace and Pablo immediately liked it. Rather than the usual dopamine hit, it made me annoyed and angry. I blocked him, and loved myself for blocking him. I had never been such a bitch, but it felt good. I had avoided anger as "bad" in the past. I wanted to stay calm and happy, not burden people with my emotions. I put Hole's *Live Through This* album in my headphones and started walking hard in angst. The setting Sun was molten copper. Cook me, transform me. I wanted to alchemize my rage into art. Making art would be the best revenge. Being mad gave me the sense of purpose I had longed for. I was not only feeling my body, I felt the strength bouncing back. My niceness had kept me muffled and scared of how people would receive me. Wanting to be liked kept me always uncertain of who I was, or who I should be. I realized it wasn't really him I was mad about, it was the deeper loss of myself that had been festering since I censored my young gay spirit. A cosmic pimple was bursting, releasing truth.

I brought white lilies to the yoga studio Easter Sunday and made an altar for the workshop. Eight people came and we shared what we intended to resurrect. I led them in the breathing pattern as they laid on blankets. The smell of the lilies filled the room. Someone started crying, releasing pent up emotion.

"Go into your heart and release any feeling of not being loved. Give yourself the Love you need, draw it in from the air, and the sunlight," I said. I felt my own heart open as I realized I wasn't alone in being hurt, in having to pick up and keep going. I felt the cosmic Jesus energy of resurrection. Maybe the kingdom was within, and you had to become like a child again? It felt triumphant to show up and lead a group even while still feeling heartbroken. I was an emotional bodybuilder getting more buff.

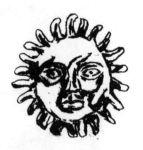

5

Venice

Dara pulled up an hour late. Her black Prius window slid open, "Baby, I'm so sorry it took forever."

"It's okay. Time is an illusion," I said. I was happy to get into the AC. We hugged and she smelled like jasmine. Her face was smooth with makeup, the texture of a soft leather handbag. Her lips were glossed in dark cherry. Dara riffed on the Disney princess archetype: goth, girlish, and elegant. We drove off and got on the 110 Freeway west towards Erewhon, the luxury health food store.

"Lukey, have you heard the new Cardi B song?"

"That stripper who became a rapper, right?"

"Yes, she's amazing. I just need you to listen to this before anything else happens."

She hit play and the bass dropped, shaking the car's speakers. Cardi mouthed accusations to a cheating boyfriend. The simplicity of the beat made space for the raw emotion in the song, and the air in the car changed as we absorbed the words: "My heart is like a package with a fragile label on it, be careful with me."

It took us an hour to get to the west side and we listened to the song on repeat as we inched through traffic.

"I feel like a female rapper has never been so emotional, femme and badass all at the same time," Dara said, watching the road.

The lyrics we obsessed most over were: "You got me looking in the mirror different. Thinking I'm flawed because you're inconsistent."

Dara and I met through the Brooklyn witch community. I was taken by both her beauty and her metaphysical mind. We shared a love for health food, fashion and complicated romances. The bubble that forms around friends as they make inside jokes and ways of talking was forming around us fast.

Dara was getting a call and turned down the music.

"It's my client, gotta take this."

She used to work at a Tantric sensual massage studio in Santa Monica but had quit and gone freelance as a geisha.

"Sure that works. I was going to come tomorrow but I can come tonight."

Dara looked like she was doing a screen test as she spoke and drove. Pouting and acting into an imaginary camera. We were in the slow lane in the last stretch of freeway before the beach. She has angular cheekbones and freckles on her nose.

Her mom is Thai and her dad is Russian Jewish. I worship her unique beauty, but it was hard for her growing up in California where the blonde Barbie look was the ideal. She'd managed to claim her beauty, though, and use it.

"Can you put the money in my account today, then? Thank you. Bless you. See you soon," she hung up and smiled at me.

"So that was my best client and he lives in Santa Barbara and I drive up there every week to see him. Feels so good to pay rent with one night. You really should get into sex work, Lukey."

We arrived at Erewhon, a supermarket where the parking is valet. Dara parked at the booth and gave the keys to a Brad Pitt lookalike who was the attendant. The parking lot looked like a luxury car dealership—Teslas, Beamers and a few other Priuses. There was a vintage Mercedes convertible with a surfboard seat-belted into the passenger seat. I felt shabby, especially with my one broken platform.

"Wait can I borrow some shoes?" I asked Dara.

She popped the trunk and I dug under yoga mats and piles of clothes to find the matching blue velvet mule sandal. They were two sizes too small and my heel hung off the back, but whatever. Heels elevate you in every way.

Erewhon is the Bergdorf's of health food. The moment the cold air hit and I walked the polished shiny concrete floors I was initiated into a new reality. The ethos here was about not just loving your body, but worshipping it. Just being there made you feel special, good, cared for.

We'd come for their drinks. The three-page menu includes herb tonic lattes, immune shots, and mint cacao protein shakes.

"I'll buy you a tonic baby. What do you want?" Dara was so generous. She was aware of the plight of her artist friends who didn't do the lucrative work she did. Things she gave me felt charged with Love and generosity. I chose their famous Jing Tonic, fifteen dollars of energy balancing herbs like deer antler and dragon bone.

We sat on the patio under a trellis of wisteria. "Where Have All the Cowboys Gone?" played from hidden speakers. "Sometimes I just come here to look for guys, because I'd know we'd have superfoods in common," Dara said, opening the compostable to-go box of lamb stew and couscous. I sipped my tonic, which was butterscotch and smoky, thanks to the Shilajit, mineral rich resin scraped off rocks in the Himalayas.

"Nice shoes," said another Brad Pitt with stubble and a trucker hat as he walked by with a tray. It felt good to be acknowledged. Fashion is a way to gain attention, just as flowers attract bees. We all seek pollination.

"How was the painting show? I'm sorry I didn't make it," Dara said, taking a bite and using her fingers to shove stems of spinach into her mouth.

"It was cool, but nothing happened between us, again. It's been a really hard few days since. When I texted him later he'd already left back to Portland. But, now that I'm here on the Westside, everything feels lifted," I said.

She shook her head with a concerned and understanding look.

It was so sunny and pretty here. The clean and healthy vibes of Venice made my dark emotions impossible to access. Within a mile radius of the beach everything gets easy-breezy. "It's so gorgeous here. Thank you for driving us!" Sitting there with her, in the wisteria's perfume, I felt deeply fulfilled. The happy vibe cleansed me of the pain I'd been feeling since Pablo's show. Maybe that's why I always sought out beauty and luxury, to counteract the heaviness and darkness of my inner world. I felt changed, but maybe it was the tonic herbs kicking in.

"Lukey, you need a guy who appreciates you. Someone who can pay. Our presence is a gift. The Yang needs to learn to honor and exchange with the Yin. You are a receptive and caring vessel, sensitive and open. They can pay. We can value the Yin, not just the Yang. Everyone thinks power is about strength and gain, but the feminine energy of The Mother absorbs, hides, and comforts. You should be getting $1000 a night. Quit worrying about these guys who don't see your beauty."

I lived for Dara's rants. They always ignited my confidence.

"Wanna go swimming at my client's apartment building?"

"Amazing, yess!" I said.

Dara used her phone as a compact to check her teeth, and then pouted and re-applied her black cherry lipstick. I copied her and checked myself out using my phone. I hadn't shaved in weeks and looked like a skinny lion with my curly hair reaching out in every direction. My chain link necklace from the hardware store hung around my neck. It was heavy, a reminder of the pain I got into chasing people who didn't love me back. I cocked my head to the side and took a photo. Dara was rubbing off on me.

It took us a long time to get to the pool at Dara's client's apartment building because the pastel bungalows of Venice captivated us. Every plant was a miracle to stroke, smell and take selfies with. The Westside of LA has more water and a sea breeze and the gardens are gently hydrated. Neither of us had even seen a jade succulent blooming before, with flowers that looked like tiny praying mantises. We weren't on drugs, but when we hung out together portals opened. Our two imaginations fused and seemed to bend reality. Dara snapped a close-up of my hairy ankle in her velvet mules. She showed me the post for approval, and I smiled. She had captioned it: "Soul Mate."

Any clothes she wore became cool because they were

touching her. Today she dressed like a celebrity in disguise: navy baseball cap embroidered with the Tesla logo, tiny sunglasses, jeans cut off at her ankles, and see-through, mule heel stripper sandals that looked like glass but were made of plastic. She brushed the screen a few times to see what else was happening around the world. Drinking up the satisfaction of likes blinking onto the screen, increasing her invisible currency.

"Lol, Elon liked it." She somehow knew important people, like the moody tech genius, she'd just message online and become friends with. The six degrees of connection to celebrities dissolved when I was with her. We were a part of that world because she said we were.

We continued walking on the peaceful Venice side street, our mule heels clicking against the cement. I wanted to bring up what I'd been reading about the goddess Inanna. I knew she would resonate and have some insight on it.

"So, you know the goddess Inanna I told you about? The myth is a road map for how to descend into the Underworld. So many light beings and New Age teachings have no references in their philosophies for how to deal with deep emotions. They just say 'think positive' but have no recommendations for how to shift the deeply held emotions that loom under the surface."

Dara nodded, "Exactly. And you're flawed if you can't just live a pretty, perfect Instagram life. If you actually have feelings, no one wants to hear them. People expect you to be either sexy or successful. When you stray and express another side of yourself, they unfollow. They want you to represent this version of life where things are simple. But sorry babes, it's not."

We both saw the rose at the same time and were left speechless by its size and clarity. Pink petals stretched wide, and a yellow bee nibbling its pollen, right at eye level. The rose abducted us into her beauty. The whole bush was dotted with them, but this one was the queen.

"Hello, Sister," Dara said, after a minute just standing there in silent awe. "We are so blessed," she said, and pulled the grapefruit sized blossom to her cheek, sighed her maroon lips open, and snapped a selfie. And then another. I hoped the house owners weren't home, watching this. She was a model and knew how to be photogenic. She looked like a rose, her skin like petals, a natural beauty.

When we got to the condos she entered the code to get in. The jellybean shaped pool was at the center of the apartments but no one was home during the week so it felt private. "Do you want some living water?" she asked.

"Ya, what's living about it?"

"It's fresh from Mount Shasta, it gets delivered every week. It's better than city water that's basically, like, dead." Maybe everything had a more alive version than I'd ever known was possible.

I jumped into the pool with my boxers and chain necklace

on. Dara didn't want to get her hair wet and gently glided in.

"I really want to be an influencer," she said. The water quivered reflections all over her. "I'm ready to be seen," she said. Something flew into her and she flinched and swatted it away. An iridescent beetle landed right on the part of her hair.

"Don't move, I have to take your picture!"

I reached for my phone and snapped her looking like a queen with this gold and purple medallion in her hair. It looked fake but it was real. Beautiful things always happened when we hung out together. "Seems like a good omen," I said.

As I pushed up out of the pool I felt like I was in a David Hockney painting, with squiggly teal water. Dara laid in the pool chair, and I laid directly on the hot stucco to dry, warming my blood. I felt so good. I was photo-synthesizing a sense of being somebody.

I spaced out and my mind expanded. I could feel the Hollywood Sign as a magic sigil, charged up by dreams and hopes. But I also felt the fear in the air. Everything has a shadow, and the shadow of wanting success was a fear of failure that caused the smog in the air. My chain had heated up and woke me up to my sweaty, roasting body.

I opened my eyes and Dara was on the pool chair with her legs bent, scrolling her phone. "What are you manifesting right now?" she asked.

I thought for a minute, and got up to sit on the pool chair

next to her. I wanted to be able to afford Erewhon every day, but I didn't want to have to sell my soul to get the money.

"I guess pursuing my passions and having enough money. And Love! Isn't everybody always wanting money and Love? So basic."

"You deserve it. Blessed be," she closed her eyes and I followed suit. We meditated for a minute, sending the prayer out from the apartment courtyard.

"What are you manifesting right now?" I asked in response.

"Influence," she said, stone faced under her Tesla cap.

"Influence over what?" I asked.

"I mean being an influencer. Having a hundred thousand followers. Getting free stuff to promote. Being important."

"It seems like it's happening for you. I love your posts."

"Thanks babe. I hope a lot more people love them, too."

We closed our eyes again to send out her prayer.

"It's all vibration," she said, after a minute of silence. I opened my eyes to her meditating, as peacefully as a rose. Her existence was always picture ready. She started channeling in meditation, tuned into a higher source. "If you believe you can have it, it will come to you. The piñata's broken open, and it's time for everyone to get their candy." Then she blinked her eyes open and went back to scrolling on her phone.

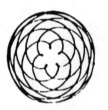

6

Malibu

I had matched with a dream guy on Tinder while packing my cabin in Woodstock. He had long hair, a chiseled body, and, as it turned out, we were both from New Mexico. I told him I was headed to LA, and magically, so was he—another synchronicity. It was a gift to have another crush since things hadn't panned out with the Painter, the original connection I'd come to LA to pursue. I kept trying to hang out with the New Mexican guy, but he was always surfing in Malibu, which only made him dreamier. "It's my spiritual practice now, the waves," he'd texted. I wanted to surf, or do anything with him. It seemed like the Universe was making up for the oversight it had made between me and the Painter by giving me another potential soul mate.

He'd been at Coachella working as a back-up dancer, and called me on his way back. He was tired, but I invited him over to just chill. On our first date he'd come over for lunch that ended in a slow make out session. He showed up a few hours later in a dirty white tank top, sunburned shoulders, tight blue jeans and a cowboy hat. We laid on the couch. "I've been tripping on LSD all weekend, I feel so fried," he said, in a deep, raspy voice. His breath smelled faintly of whiskey. The narrow couch forced us to squeeze tightly. He was so warm, my nervous system relaxed in his arms. "You should charge people to cuddle with you," I said. He laughed.

The air from his laugh on my neck made me twitch because I'm very ticklish. He thought that was funny and kept laughing to torture me. Then we fell asleep. When I woke up in a soft daze I ran my fingers through his hair. He reminded me of Legalas, the hot elf in *Lord of the Rings*. He seemed out of my league. I'm more of a Hobbit with fairy DNA. My Mom's Scottish ancestors supposedly married into the Faeries. My Dad's side are Russian Jews. I'm not sure which side gives me coarse brown hair everywhere, down to my toe knuckles, but I hoped this guy was into Hobbits.

This is what I had longed for. Body heat and whispers. I have wanted a Love like John and Yoko's ever since I saw the photo of them entwined in my babysitter's room. I've known since kindergarten that to be naked in a fetal position, wrapped in someone's long hair is what I am here for. The difficulties of life would be bearable with someone to cuddle with through it. As I held him, I started feeling some Golem energy creep in, the villain whose greed drives him crazy. I could feel how I would never want to share him if we became a couple. I held him like the precious gold ring.

"My precious," I said as I stroked his hair.

"What?" he asked confused as he woke up.

"Don't ever cut your hair," I said.

A second date should be epic. It says, "hey, you passed the first test, now I want to show you how good this could be." It is also before you can see any of the challenges you might face.

"I wanna take you camping in Malibu someday," he said. His breath tickled my neck again.

"When do you leave again?"

"Tomorrow at noon."

Suddenly I realized this couch moment would end. Our body heat on the fabric would cool. The couch would hold other people, and so would we.

"We can probably still beat traffic if we leave now," he said. "Can you pack in like, three minutes? I can take you to the airport tomorrow morning."

His eyes were glossy as he waited for my response. I slid off the couch and packed chaotically. Whatever I left behind would be worth sacrificing for getting to be with him for my last night in LA. I rolled my suitcase out of the bedroom. He stood up and rubbed his eyes sleepily. I could see his banana shaped dick print in his blue jeans. His hotness made me feel wobbly.

We made it under the overpasses of downtown without stopping. "We did it, we beat traffic!" he said, grabbing my thigh with his hand. I reached to massage his neck and shoulders. The Sun was blasting into the car, dust particles shimmered in the air. This was what I'd been manifesting. My life coach had guided me in making affirmations and visualizations to prime my subconscious for what I wanted. This was the first image I'd come up with, driving with a guy and he grabs my thigh. "My life is fabulously fulfilling," was the affirmation I'd come up with to match the visual. It was like realizing a Ouija board worked. Magic was real. My affirmations and images had manifested this into reality. I was a verified wizard.

"I have to make a call to my friend about the piece we're choreographing in Mexico," he said, unaware of the life changing experience I was going through. I nodded and snapped a photo of his hand on my leg to send to my life coach. The highway was flowing, and for the first time, I wished there was traffic. I wanted to be trapped forever in this moment. There was a stick of palo santo in the ashtray and I lit it and watched the blue smoke billow. The sharp woody aroma matched the mystical mood I was in. Thank you Goddess, I prayed, as we passed between hills and the light flickered in the smoky air.

We merged onto the Pacific Coast Highway and the ocean sparkled out the window. He was playing surf rock, lots of Angel Olsen. Making it to the edge of a city was always a relief, like reaching the finish line of Earth. Heaven and hell are states of mind, and I wanted to never fall from this level of bliss again. I tried to stay in the moment and just enjoy it. We stopped at a grocery store for firewood and food to grill. He seemed to have this camping trip to Malibu down to a science, did he take all his second dates here? As I pumped gas, I wondered if we could keep this flame alive.

We got to the campground at dusk and he set up the tent. It quickly got chilly so we made a fire, then stared at the flames in silence. Sitting on the edge of the fire pit, we started kissing. The only sound was sparking wood and wet lips. My stomach grumbled. We stopped and laughed. "I guess somebody's hungry?" he said.

He pulled out his box of utensils and we used the paper bag as a cutting board. Once we got the peppers, zucchinis, and chicken breasts on the grill, I grabbed my guitar from the car to serenade him. He watched over the fire with his cowboy hat and jean jacket on. I sang, "Strong Enough to Be My Man" by Sheryl Crow, and one of my own songs that I rarely shared with anyone. I stared at the flames as I strummed the last chord. He didn't say anything. The cicadas hummed and the fire crackled. Were the songs too sentimental? I couldn't read what he was feeling. I should have asked, but I wanted to play it cool and just have fun.

After dinner we walked to the beach under the highway

through a corrugated metal tunnel. It was windy and cold. There were no stars and the green tinge of light pollution from LA gave an eerie sense of what we had gotten away from for the night. We laid down on the yoga blanket he'd brought and squeezed together.

"Don't worry I'll keep you warm, I'm exothermal," he said.

"What does that mean?" I asked.

"I give off a lot of heat."

We were so well matched, I thought, because my hands and feet were always cold.

It was the New Moon and I wanted to set intentions with him. I had planned this before we left camp, putting two dimes in my pocket. "You wanna make New Moon intentions? The energy is potent for it," I said. We stood up and walked to the edge of the water.

"I'll go first. My intention is to turn pain into art," I threw my dime out but didn't hear it plop over the loud static of the wind on the waves.

"I'm wishing for the possibilities to turn into something," he said and tossed it in.

I wondered if he meant the possibility of me, but I didn't want to ask and ruin his wish.

Then he picked me up and pretended to throw me in the ocean and I screamed.

When we got back to the tent we started kissing by the

fire again. It was dying down and spewed charcoal-smelling smoke. We made our way to the tent, pausing to explore newly exposed parts of our bodies as we undressed each other. We made it to the two-person sleeping bag. I noted the fact that owning a two-person sleeping bag meant he must often share it with people, but hey, it was me tonight. My mind grasped as the pleasure started to take over. Am I good enough? Does he really like me? The sensations weren't as strong when I was distracted by thoughts. I had to surrender to the feeling. And when I did it was overwhelming.

We were opening a Tantric portal. Gays don't make babies but our sex creates something. It felt like we had dimension-hopped to a Heavenly realm, where the pain of Earth was healed by eroticism. The nylon swiped as we rolled around. The tent was steamed up from our body heat. As he pounded me I grunted and coyotes started howling outside. Maybe they were fucking too. We both pushed over the edge and orgasmed, life force charging through our bodies. "Oh shit!" he said and we jizzed like two shooting stars streaking through the sky. We paused in the charged silence. Then he grabbed a bandana to wipe up our juices before spooning me in the sleeping bag. His hair spread around us on the pillow.

I unzipped the tent the next morning to the sunny campsite. I picked up my plaid boxers, and followed the trail of strewn clothes back to the fire pit, getting dressed along the way. He emerged naked from the tent and stretched his arms up. "Let's pack and then go swimming to rinse off. Then we can stop for coffee," he said.

"Sounds perfect."

"You're perfect," he said, giving me a peck.

I breathed in the dry grass and purple dirt hills to help me remember this place forever. While carrying the sleeping bag to the car, I saw a flash reflected in the ground. I bent down and picked up a diamond out of the gravel. I examined its pyramid point and faceted top. It must have fallen out of someone's wedding ring. I thought it was a good omen for romance. I told him that as we drove away and we laughed. "I'm gonna leave this with you. If it's real it's worth a lot, so you should get it checked!" I said, dropping it in his ashtray.

"This is my favorite swimming beach," he said as we pulled off a random spot on the PCH. There were no signs or other cars around. I borrowed his red Speedo and he wore his boxer briefs and cowboy hat and we scaled the cliff down to the water barefoot. The water was sharply cold but it felt good to rinse off. I sat on the shore and shivered in a towel as he floated like an otter above the waves to keep his hat dry. I wanted every morning to be like this. We got back in the car and drove a few minutes down the coast to a coffee shop on a pier. There were pick-ups with surfboards hanging out the back and wetsuits hanging to dry. I appreciated that he had given us enough time to enjoy some more magic in the morning.

As we got closer to the airport, he told me his dad had been a wanderer and had been in and out of his family growing up. I could feel the sadness and lostness he'd inherited. He had the freedom of a wanderer but also the nihilism of learning not to hold on. His eyes looked extra watery again, like a mermaid out of water. When we pulled up to the airport he got my suitcase out of the trunk. "Call me sometime," he said, taking off his cowboy hat to give me a kiss goodbye.

I reluctantly checked in, I didn't want to leave when a romance was just starting . An hour into the plane ride, my bones still chilled and hair damp, I decided to move to LA full time. My corduroy jacket reeked of campfire. The scent was a reminder of the magic we'd made. I hoped it would never fade.

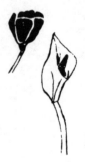

7
Divine Timing

I went back to Brooklyn for the month of May to pack. I imagined Ballet Surfer would meet me at the airport and we'd pick up where we'd left off. But while I closed my life in NYC, he stopped responding. It was disheartening, but he wasn't the only reason I was going to LA. Wanting a new chapter I released nearly all my belongings. From my third-floor window in Fort Greene, I could see people browsing my free books on the stoop downstairs. Having found so much stuff on the street in New York, it felt good to give back.

When I arrived at LAX, I still thought Ballet Surfer might surprise me, but he didn't so I took a cab. Some things manifest so easily, while others remain stubbornly out of reach. I still hadn't met a partner, but I had good real estate luck. I had wanted to live in a house just like Ruby's, with friends, on the Eastside. In May, Ruby told me his roommate Shane was looking for someone to sublet his room. He'd quit his barista job to spend the summer camping. And so it aligned perfectly that I landed at Ruby's house.

Traffic was light, and it only took thirty minutes to get to the Eastside. In New York you are part of a crowd, in LA you are part of traffic. I passed a '60s car with fins and chrome, keeping the Route 66 Americana style alive.

The house was on Dexter, a steep road in Highland Park. The street was narrow and was lined with parallel parked cars. We passed more vintage cars, and a shiny black lowrider. When we arrived, I dead lifted my suitcase full of crystals up steep stairs leading to the door. The house looked like a kid's drawing: square with a pitched roof and the sunshine in the upper right corner. There were three huge agave plants in front, a fruiting lemon tree, a lavender bush, bougainvillea, and cacti. As I opened the gate, hanging chimes tinkled and announced my arrival. Shane came outside, shading his eyes with his hand. "Welcome buddy! Come on in, I'll give you a tour," he said.

He looked like a Peter Pan lost boy—barefoot, in cut off shorts with visible ribs. He grew up in Santa Barbara and had that golden Cali warmth to him.

His stuff was monastically organized and tucked away to make space for me. He'd put a lily in an old kombucha bottle on the desk. The bed was on top of wood shipping pallets and felt like hardened clay. I liked his DIY vibe. The window was covered in overgrown ivy and couldn't be opened, but the ivy created a natural blind to the neighbor's backyard. The French doors opened to the patio, and on a hot night you could sleep with them open, Shane said.

He put on his backpack; it was taller than him. He looked like an ant carrying a potato. His tin pan and mug clanked as we hugged. "I left the electric guitar out for you to jam on," he said. I saw the watercolor outline of the mountains where he was headed in the distance as he walked away down the stairs. Not a day went by that I wasn't grateful to him for giving me an easeful landing in LA.

Over the following week, I continued the same routine I'd had in New York: wake up, drink a glass of water, meditate for ten minutes, then go get a double espresso and journal. Cafe de Leche was at the bottom of the hill. My walk there each morning became sacred, because it was the only time of day when I knew where I was going: to get coffee. The rest of the day I was completely lost and confused. I got to know the plants in the neighborhood, breathing in the rosemary as I passed the yard full of it. The San Gabriel Mountains were usually blurred by smog, but would come into sharp and clear focus when it rained. I learned to cross the street to avoid setting off three cocker spaniels that always barked. In the morning life is fresh with new potentials and familiar annoyances.

Time felt different in LA. People didn't have the sense of urgency they did in New York, something that stood out at the cafe when I was fiending for caffeine. In LA, people have drawn out conversations with baristas before they order.

"So what are you doing on your day off?"

"Probably hiking in Ojai."

"Oh, I'm from there. Where are you going hiking?"

One morning in my second week, the barista puts down the paper cup and leans on the counter to chat. I want to interject and say, "can you please multi-task? Like, work while you chat?" Instead I stand there impatiently, recalling cafes in New York where you have five seconds to deliver your order before they skip on to the next person. As the girl in front of me decides she wants her coffee iced instead of hot, I think about how scenes and experiences are mirrors for us, and how the way we react to them often shows us something about ourselves. I wonder, am I too sped up from my years in the city?

Once I order my coffee, I face the headlines of the New York Times they keep on the counter. I am relieved when the news is not shocking, and not surprised when it is. As I scan the calamities, lies and injustice, the bean grinder roars and the steam wand hisses. I'm so thankful for the machine extracting this stimulant; coffee is what I need to jumpstart my life. It gives me an artificial drive. Even if you don't know where you're going, on caffeine at least you're going there fast. As I grab my mason jar of coffee, the barista compliments my jacket and we talk about the local thrift stores for a minute before she gets back to the line that's now out the door.

Sometimes I journal in the cafe, but that day I walk back up the hill, waiting to take my first sip 'til I am at the patio table with my journal and pen. I write as a meditation. "I felt so light leaving New York, but now I spend my time wondering what to desire and where to go. Trying to find the magnetic pull within."

Once my brain is drained of emotions, I turn my phone on. The only thing worse than getting a difficult text in the morning is getting no texts at all. I feel the same familiar sense of betrayal every day Ballet Surfer doesn't text. I shut my phone off and restart it just in case.

Then Ruby comes out the front door dressed for a 1980s prom: white button-down shirt, black pants, and Ray Ban sunglasses. Fresh and dewy from his Plato skin care routine, he makes me want to look as smooth and groomed as he is. But is it the products, or just the radiance of who he is? "Good morning Young Skywalker," he says with a bow. "My manager said you can bring in your resume, by the way."

I take a beat to imagine myself working there, my hair slicked back, leaving at 10:15am in case there was traffic. I could still walk to the cafe and write every morning. "Great news. Thanks for asking her. I hope you have a good day at work, bud."

We do gun hands at each other and he walks off with a

bounce in his step. Once I hear the chimes of the gate, I know I am alone for the day. The other roommate Calvin is a massage therapist who leaves before I wake up to beat the traffic to his office in Beverly Hills.

I lie out in the Sun. At least I am working on my tan. To the drones that pass every 30 minutes on the same route, I must be cataloged as just another unemployed mystic. But what the drones can't see is that I am hacking the mystery of reality. I am reading *The Holographic Universe* for the second time, slowly because the science jargon is so confusing. If I could just figure out how to crack the hologram maybe I wouldn't have to get a real job?

I would strum chord progressions at the patio table but my lyrics were cliché and I couldn't finish songs. I wanted to make my music different; why do something that has been done before? I felt the same pressure to innovate in my healing work, and didn't think I was good enough yet to really promote it. I laid there with the cacti and the passionflower bush, the slowness was making me panic. I should be doing something, getting somewhere. Intellect is tricky; it can help you understand your place in the cosmos, but it can also tangle you in confusion. I was trying to accept that the Universe isn't a vending machine that gives you whatever you want when you want it and be patient.

I saw friends who were healers growing big followings

and becoming famous. I felt pressure to make something that I could sell, so I could make a living off of it. When I posted YouTube videos of myself talking about spiritual topics no one watched. Maybe I wasn't excited enough about the topic to engage people? To be successful would mean having to appeal to a mass audience, and that meant I would not be able to express myself freely. Were the two things really mutually exclusive?

I posted a shirtless selfie and then deleted it. I wanted to use Instagram as a place to share my healing work *and* meet lovers, a hard balance to strike. I saw how people on social media became so one dimensional: "I'm Katie the Healer!" All she thinks about is healing? Really? She restricts herself to one topic and a color scheme. Being a brand feels so overly self-conscious. I wanted to be free, unashamed to share all parts of me, and to share that spirituality was personal, unique and didn't have to look any one way.

I took out my journal and make a pros and cons list of working a normal job. Then I got up to take my resume to both Plato and Venus Juice.

That weekend, Alexandra invited me to New Age church with her. She was a famous healer on Instagram whose authenticity and writing I loved. She embraced the gritty, sexy and magical sides of being human. She texted: "Let's go to New Age church

Sunday at Agape. It's not a cult, it's amazing." We arrived at 8:45am on Sunday morning to a huge building in Culver City that used to be a TV studio. The shuffle of everyone arriving at church, dressed up and courteous, was heart-warming. It was beautiful right away to be in such a diverse community: all races and ages. Whatever it was that was bringing so many different people together was something I wanted to partake in.

The service began with a guided meditation. The leader, Reverend Michael, was a radiant Black man wearing sneakers and a blazer. As he started preaching, a mix of classical church and new age spirituality, my heart began opening. "It's time to wake up, old souls! If you've been slumbering, caught up in the dream of materialism and consumerism, it's time to wake up and realize your needs are met from the inside out. Find your gifted area and express it more completely, profoundly, more consistently," he told us. People in the audience called out in support: "Amen!"

The Agape band was playing, and they grooved into a set of ballads sung by a Priestess with long braids and necklaces of Rudraksha beads. "Use me, use me Lord, fill my heart with Pure Agape Love," she sang. The band vamped, filling the large cavernous room with soul-shaking sound, and Reverend Michael said: "If it's your first time to Agape please stand up. We are so happy you are here."

Alexandra elbowed me with a smile and I stood. Everyone around smiled at me and made prayer hands. Reverend Michael continued to address us new folks: "You are a light, you are a gift, you are a part of God and we are glad you are here. We see you. We see you. We know your greatness. Bless you." I blushed from getting so much attention. I didn't know how much I'd needed this encouragment.

A room full of 500 people feeling the same Love and devotion has an intense empathic effect. I felt a welling of emotions like at the end of a movie when the good guys just won. When the Priestess started her last song, "The Spirit of God is Upon Me," I lost it. Her voice carried so much emotion, I could feel the triumph of what she'd been through to get to her spiritual healing in the depth and range of her vocals. The words were about finding your own authentic spirituality: "I used to think that I had to. I used to think that I should. Because the Bible told me that I had to be good. But now I Love 'cause I want to. I Love because I am free. Grateful for the Spirit, oh Lord, the Spirit of God is upon me."

The Spirit in the room, all those hearts opening, combined with the throbbing bass, the background chorus ... I started bawling. It was totally unexpected; I hadn't felt especially sad before, but the healing energy in the room pressed something out of me that was beyond my control. I gasped and the tears burned. The salt and sadness from Malibu was coming out. It felt like being tumbled in a laundry cycle of Love. I felt connected to God, and trusted that I had been brought here for a reason and that I was still on the right track. I could feel the divine timing I was a part of.

After the catharsis of the song ended, I was trembling. The tithing baskets went out and I gave twenty dollars but wished I could have given a thousand. I was so moved and thankful. The experience reminded me that, just as easy as it is for me to feel romantic Love, or existential doom, I am also open to the unseen energetic forces of Spirit that heal. I remembered that to feel a lot is also a gift. Being an empath and an Indigo has liabilities, but I just had to remember to reach for the good to stay on track.

After church we went to Cafe Gratitude.

The patio was like a wedding reception: white napkins and chairs. Our other friends who had been at church, but seated separately, Sah and Moun, joined us for brunch. All four of us were healers and it was fun to all be on the same page. Everyone was fully charged from church.

I ordered the "I Am Fulfilled" kelp noodles and the "I am Immortal" immunity latte. Somehow, the first topic we hit on was my disappointment about Ballet Surfer not working out. I had come back down to Earth from my Agape high. Back to whining! They were also all life coaches and I needed a triple-threat teamwork session to process this.

"Why do you keep attracting this unrequited energy into

your life?" Sah asked, sipping his "I Am Awake" matcha latte.

"I know I am a soul. I want to feel the infinity of every moment, but there is another side of me that is so broken," I said, and started to cry again, the Agape emotions still churning.

"You deserve more," Alexandra told me, her bangles clanking as she lovingly patted my leg. "Is that a menu option?" Sah asked gregariously. "Can we order 'I deserve more,' whether it's a salad or whatever?" We laughed, which made me cry again.

As we ate, the conversation shifted onto our projects and work. Moun was leading her first retreat and going back to practice meditation in India. I shared that I was hoping to get the job at the Juice Shop. "Okay, I get it, you want the stability, but just remember you are next lev-el, honey. Don't you forget it," Sah said, tossing his hair over his other shoulder as punctuation. I loved being with them because they inspired me to reach and believe in myself.

That night I got a message from someone on Schlong who I recognized from Tinder. "What does it mean when you match on two different dating apps?" I asked. "That we're both desperate?" they responded.

We made a date to meet the next day in Echo Park. Sigil had black nails, long black hair, a beanie and converse high tops. They had grown up in LA, and were an intriguing mix of masculine and femme energies. On the first date, I learned Sigil used she/they pronouns. We started going through all the requisite interview questions for a first date. We were briefly interrupted by the bell of an ice cream pushcart. Sigil unwrapped the popsicle and bit off its head. "So, what do you think my sign is?" Melted ice cream was dripping down their black nails. I don't really like to talk astrology until I've gotten to know someone. It's better when you know someone first and then figure out their signs, rather than to project all your ideas about the signs on them right away.

But fuck it. They had to be Scorpio. "How did you know?!" "Well, you're deep, intriguing, have black nails, are witchy and sexy." Neither of us could help but indulge in diving fully into our connection. Rather than suss it out and let it grow over time, we completed three months of dating in one afternoon.

Sigil and I went on a few more dates after that. By noon the June gloom clouds would burn off, and we'd sunbathe on my patio naked. Massaging one another with coconut oil. When we got hungry, I had to admit my dwindling savings: "I gotta save money, let's cook at home." It was that point in dating when you can't hide your problems anymore. I felt too overwhelmed by my money and career problems to hold space for someone else. I started to pull away, fearing we'd spin into drama quickly. The last time we hung out Sigil gave me an abundance spell candle, just in time for the Capricorn Full Moon. I'd never dated another witch. It felt like they had charged it up with intention. "I could tell you needed to do some magic," she said when she gave it to me.

That night, I went outside to see the cat-eye Moon rise above the lemon tree. The neighborhood dogs howled at it. I wished for work and money for my new life in LA, struck the match, and lit the candle. The wax smelled like jasmine. I let it burn in my room over the next few days. Even though me and Sigil didn't work out, the connection we'd shared gave me excitement and support to take the next step. I hope I did the same in return for them.

The next day, I got a call from Venus Juice. I had an interview Friday. I took a Lyft to the Melrose Place location to meet the manager, Lacy. She had a blonde bob, a Southern lilt and wore twinkling diamond jewelry. I had never thought a manager could be so charming and kind. At the end of our chat under the white umbrella on the sidewalk of the Juice Shop, she offered me the job.

I rolled the car windows down in my ride-share on the way home and breathed in the Friday morning air. I sipped the iced chai with mood boosting mushrooms Lacy had made me for the road. It felt like a rainbow after the storm. The job lifted a huge weight, as now I would have a steady source of income. It had been a frustrating transition, but I could see how it had unfolded in divine timing. The job gave me a sense of purpose. I didn't realize how much I'd needed it until I had it back. Even if it was just a juice shop, I had to be somewhere Monday.

8

The Juice Shop

The Juice Shop has been called a cult. Regulars come in daily and don't take off their sunglasses. There are celebrity sightings, and that raises the status of the brand. This is a new type of luxury wellness. The rainbow of juices quench thirst, boost immunity, and detoxify. My new job included taste-testing the juices daily, offering samples to everyone who walked in the door and sharing my passion for the natural beauty products we sold. I was drinking the left-over green juice, living the LA dream.

It started with two weeks of rigorous training. I had to taste all the juices and learn how to describe them, like a wine sommelier. We had juices of every color: maroon beet, emerald spinach, and pink strawberry almond milk. Then there were the herbs, sold in small glass jars with doodled labels. I had to learn all about the benefits and what to recommend for different ailments. I liked the witchy aspect of the job. It wasn't far off from the healing sessions I had been offering people. Except rather than meditation and energy work, now I'd just recommend the jar best suited to them.

Tara, who'd served me the first time I came to the shop after bumping into Oz at The House of Intuition, became my teacher. She had pink tinted hair and kind eyes. We would arrive at 6:30am, the refrigerators snoring loudly. Tara wore a baggy Mickey Mouse sweatshirt until the shop warmed up. The uniform was either all white or blue jeans. We were provided with white aprons.

The store's decor was minimal and clean, with large potted plants on the floor like a Japanese garden on a spaceship. There was a sense of takeoff and landing in the daily routine. Cesar was waiting in his pickup when we arrived with the daily delivery of fresh juice from the main kitchen. There was a detailed checklist of tasks to complete every shift. Right on schedule, at 7am I checked off "put juices away," and "unlock door." I got a sense of clarity and simplicity from this daily routine.

My first real customer was a thin blonde woman on a two-week juice cleanse. "How have you been feeling on the cleanse?" Tara asked her. "I was really hungry so I broke down and had some crackers. But feeling lighter and energized," she replied. The woman was a fitness trainer and I could see the precision and control in her upright posture and tense neck. There was an undercurrent of diet culture in the Juice Shop. "I want something light. Can I see the nutrition facts?" customers would sometimes ask. The wellness culture in LA was supposed to be about helping people feel good and be healthier, but sometimes this just meant being thin. It's a fine line between narcissism and self-love.

I looked back to my list of tasks: it was time to "turn on music" and "check for expired products." The soundtrack was curated seasonally by a DJ whose psychedelic electronica fit the spaceship feel. I flipped over every product in the front fridge to double check for "spills," our code for products that were past their expiration date and that would have to be thrown out. The owner believed in the increased bioavailability of raw food, and her commitment to not pasteurizing made the product high quality but very perishable. The three-day shelf life made for a quick turn over, and we followed the food service maxim FIFO—first in, first out—to minimize waste and profit loss. "Remember to FIFO the front fridge, put the new ones in the back," Tara yelled as I put away today's fresh juice.

"I found two chia puddings that expired," I told Tara, back in the office where she was counting her cash drawer. "Oh great, we can each have one." The best part of the job was that we had access to the spills. We always started with a small taste in case it had turned. "I love pairing chia pudding with California Sun," Tara said, as we sipped sample cups of the grapefruit and orange juice.

Our next task was to sample the juices that came in today

and rate them for taste, color and packaging. I couldn't believe I was drinking all this Venus Juice for free, and getting paid. But in the last days of my training, I realized the company wasn't as chill as the packaging would have you believe.

I was feeling more confident in my role, and Tara and I had become good friends. We were blown away by how good the Canyon Greens was that morning. Was the celery more salty? Or the kale more sweet? In the "tasting notes" section, where we were supposed to write something like "not enough mint," I suggested we make a haiku. We counted the syllables and composed this:

Ginger lemon clouds
Over leafy green mountains
Delicious morning

We joyfully submitted the email before the morning rush began at 8:30am. When the phone rang, Tara said it was for me. It was Kimberly. I was confused about why the supervisor would be calling me, and immediately got scared and tingly. "Hi Luke, it's Kimberly. I know you are doing your best at learning the Venus culture, but the email you just sent was not appropriate. You might be creative on your outside time, but on the floor, we need you to be a juice professional. The owner, the president, the CEO, CFO, and myself, all read this email daily. Not to mention the kitchen staff, who are mostly ESL and may not understand your humor. We think you are a good fit for the company and I wanted to be clear about this going forward."

This was a common reaction to my creative expression, the kind I'd gotten all my life. So while it made me want to cry, as if once again I was too weird, and would never find a place to express myself, I replied in a diplomatic way. "Thanks for letting me know Kimberly. It won't happen again."

Reprimanding boss,
She doesn't deserve haiku,
Cold morning at work

I paused in the office and counted the syllables for a better last line. "Luke, I need you," Tara yelled. The rush had started. I would have to figure it out on my lunch break. Back at the counter, the blenders shredded and I steamed coconut milk for matchas that would be sipped as our customers sat in traffic.

Kimberly visited the shops regularly to do quality control. Her job was to notice what was wrong in the shop, or with the employees at any moment. She looked like the owner, with long hippie hair, and a skinny body in tight jeans. She showed up later that morning, as we washed the blenders and sponged down the counters from the rush.

Watching us work, she said, "It looks really untidy back there."

"We just had a huge rush," Tara said.

"Okay, well as a customer, I wouldn't know that, and this is what I would be seeing when I arrived."

She opened the refrigerator and pulled out three small turmeric shot bottles, cracked the lids off and gulped them quickly. Then she reached for three vitamin gel packets, tore them open, and dragged them through her teeth. She washed the egg tasting gel down with a vial of mineralizing ocean water. This all happened in under thirty seconds, like she was training for the juice Olympics. She saw us watching her. "Sorry, I haven't had any shots today and my inflammation has been flaring up." She wore a blue tie-dyed ascot around her neck to cover a pink, peeling rash. She rang up the thirty-dollar wellness binge and zeroed it out as a manager comp.

Kimberly was taking notes on a clipboard, making sure the shop was in order. The sample tray was full of tasting cups of vegan cookie dough and the curated soundtrack was playing at a reasonable volume. But then, "Oh my god. Have these bottles been backwards all day?" We turned juices backwards at night that will be expiring the next day; it was another system we do daily to track inventory and avoid spoilage.

I stared at her, paralyzed, as I watched her face contort

and turn pink. "Did you forget to take your Brain Dust today? Oh no, don't tell me, you've never even tasted Brain Dust. You should do a green juice cleanse for brain fog, too. I don't want an excuse, I just want you to fix it so the logo faces our customers when they arrive. I'm putting this in your store notes to corporate with your name on it."

Kimberly's rash was overflowing beyond her ascot. It looked like chicken pox. I could tell she lived in her own self-critical hell. She did another round of shots to calm the inner inflammation. During one of my training sessions, she'd shared that she had an auto-immune disorder that had led her to change her diet and rely on food as medicine. I wasn't sure if diet alone could cure all our problems. But, the elegant and quasi-clinical branding gave a sense of support and peace along the way, and made you feel you were taking care of yourself.

I wanted to lay Kimberly down and put my hand on her heart and for us to take some deep breaths together. I couldn't turn off my healer side. I wanted to let her know she didn't have to be abusive to be powerful. But I also didn't want to cross a boundary, so I just said, "I'm sorry, Kimberly, it will never happen again."

The job was helping me see myself in a fresh and clear light. When I started at the Juice Shop I thought I'd give up on being a healer. It was a chapter in my life that hadn't panned out. But, being there I accepted part of me is naturally a healer. I want the best for people, and want to help them. I've always been sensitive and can feel people's emotions empathically. In energy work sessions I had the ability to navigate a conversation towards what wanted to be revealed, engaging people in questions based on what I felt coming up. But I also knew I needed to do more of my own inner work. It was too easy for me to take on other people's stuff while I hadn't built up a strong enough sense of who I was.

Talking with hundreds of people a day at the Juice Shop was helping me regain my energetic boundary. I learned how to come back into my own vibe by walking and jamming to the music on my headphones on my breaks. I would walk up and down Sunset to get fish tacos, releasing other people's energy by getting my blood flowing, the movement of my physical body, and the joy music brings. I was learning that life puts you in the right situations to learn what you need next on your path.

My favorite customers proved that my dreams of LA were real. There were four regulars I called "The Beach Boys." They were surfer friends and were always freshly sun-kissed with sunglasses that resembled, in both shape and color, 1960s cars. With regular customers you learn about each other drip-by-drip, visit-by-visit. We pieced together their story: they lived together, surfed, and worked for different art and fashion companies. They seemed to have zero troubles in the world. Except for one time, when one of the Beach Boys came in with an appalled face. He'd been stuck in traffic for two and a half hours driving back to the Eastside after surfing. I suggested a dose of Spirit Dust. Traffic is one of the worst stressors in LA. But otherwise, these guys seemed to skim the waves of life. I wondered how they did it. They had no confidence issues or doubts, and seemed to seize the joy and fulfillment of every moment.

I saw this quality often in men in LA: laid back, confident, unencumbered. It wasn't that they didn't care, more that they seemed to have found a balance between their bodies and the world around them. Not like the sensitive people, who needed herbs and diets to balance their health and learn how to live in the world. The Beach Boy types I saw dotted around LA seemed chill, at ease with life. It actually seemed they might have no shadow. That they were that simple. Would that ever be possible for me?

Another regular was a DJ with a Friday night radio show of dance music from around the world. He drove a convertible Mercedes and often visited Morocco and Paris, where he'd split his time growing up. One day I was talking to my gay co-worker Jacques about who the hottest customers were and he described him and had nick-named him Moroccan Daddy. He had a Cesar haircut with salt and pepper hair, and wore '80s Adidas tracksuits and a gold chain. Sometimes he would come in sweaty after playing soccer. His girlfriend was younger than me, and his jokes were sharp and dirty without being mean or awkward. Moroccan Daddy was the only customer I would not begrudge for coming in five minutes before we closed to order an elaborate smoothie. I enjoyed his company and didn't mind doing all the dishes again, just for him, knowing I was keeping him juiced.

And then there was the guy we named Juice Daddy—a tan, blonde dad of a toddler. He drove a black Range Rover with tinted windows and always brought insulated reusable lunch boxes. We were his grocery store. He brought a shopping list. When I was first starting it was stressful, too fast and complicated: "three Strawberry Clouds, four almond unsweetened milks from the back, the 'latest dates' (freshest) you have." He was fastidious—checking the expiration dates, and the receipt, making sure he was charged correctly. He was also important because he would always drop $200, and the company looked at our averages each day. We aimed for $30 per customer (two juices and a snack, say). Therefore, if people are coming in for one $10 juice, your average dropped, and you needed a big sale to pull it back up. This encouraged us to upsell—what snack was really good with that juice, grab this for later, you'll surely be thirsty again. Juice Daddy was always my angel because my average soared after ringing up his ticket. We were friends except that he intimidated me. He was warm and seemed easy going but there was a precision to him—you knew he could be a dick if you rubbed him the wrong way. But that edge also made him kind of sexy. It was complicated.

"See if this card works, it's Canadian" he said one time. I slid it into the computer—$160 of juice, nut balls, and rose dusted chocolates. "My family came here in the Gold Rush from Canada. We were some of the first white people here. Some of us still use the old banks in Canada." The history of California flashed before my eyes: Native Americans, mountains, virgin rivers, gold panning, settlers, robbery, cowboys, civilization, blood, gold floating in hands, 1920s Hollywood, Model T cars, fur stoles, cigarettes on long holders, muscle men posing in striped shorts.

"All good, right?" he asked, breaking my daydream, saluting me and heading out the door.

I saw the old-timey opportunist pioneer in him. The gold digger who'd come to this beautiful land. Whose land was it really?

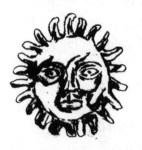

9
The Lexus

With my first paycheck I bought a car. I had always wanted a '96 Lexus like my Aunt Bee had. The leather smelled fancy and the AC was icy. I test drove a few on Craigslist. One was a low rider, and during the test drive I kept scraping speed bumps and driveways. Another located by the LA River had peeling paint and torn leather seats. It was mostly gold, with one navy door, and a copper hood. It had been patch-worked from a scrap car after a fender bender, the grandma selling it told me. The condition would have frightened most, but for me, it was perfection. The half-broken and lived-in are the honest things of life. I love hand-me-downs with rips and missing buttons. It's worth more to me when something has history.

As I drove away from the grandma's, I thought the car needed a maiden voyage and maybe if I drove to Malibu I'd run into Ballet Surfer. He had mentioned he sometimes lived at that campground—the one we'd slept at—for weeks on end. It had been four months since he ghosted me. I had tried to move on, but I was still hoping he'd text back and tell me the diamond we found on our date was real. I decided to go back. I could just sleep in my car and enjoy the beach if nothing else. I put my comforter in the trunk and hit the road feeling lucky.

The car's bells and whistles, twenty years later, had become finicky. It was too late to get my twelve hundred dollars back as I discovered everything wrong with the car. I was trying to accept the wabi-sabi of both my life and the car; the perfect imperfection. Whether it was the grandma's lingering energy, or the personality of the car, I felt calm and patient driving the Lexus. I usually drive like I'm playing Grand Theft Auto, weaving at high speed. But in the Lexus I could just be here now in traffic. I was excited to have a cassette player and had brought my tote bag of tapes.

I put in Sade's *Diamond Life*, which seemed appropriate for the Lexus. The bass line of "Paradise" started and then sped up into chipmunk sounds. I tried another tape, and listened to an entire Spice Girls song in 15 seconds. I tried not to be disappointed, it was just another thing in my life to love unconditionally. At least the radio still worked. It was on the oldies station when I bought it, so I put it back and never changed it, in honor of Grandma Ramona. I passed the heart shaped bougainvillea on the side of the highway; this must be a good sign that I was going to find him. Maybe we'd surf.

Light glittered off the ocean on the Pacific Coast Highway. "Roll all the windows down," the cliffs psychically told me. That's when I discovered only my window worked. Again, I tried not to be disappointed, but grateful—at least I had the window that mattered the most. I breathed in the salty air. Wind was blowing strong, messing up my hair. A jangly Beatles song with harmonica came on and I turned it all the way up: "and when I ask you to be my-ine, you're gonna say you love me too." I couldn't wait to take off his cowboy hat and kiss his freckled shoulders.

I pulled into the campground, but the ranger at the gate told me they were full. My plan had failed, I was angry at the campers for cock blocking me. I made a U-turn and then stopped at a scenic overlook where he might see me if he drove by.

I thought he'd feel my vibe and be psychically drawn to me. It was so fluid the times we'd hung out. Why didn't he want it to happen again? I sat on the hood of my car facing the ocean and opened the gay sex app Schlong on my phone. I scrolled through but he wasn't online. Was it my intuition that led me here, or delusional longing? I didn't feel beachy now. I realized how loud the six-lane highway was and the waves were chaotic, uninviting. My brain was doing the math: why didn't he want me, divided by what had I done wrong, times what could I do to get him back? The ocean roar and flying motors droned in a loud static, like a particle accelerator. I felt my atoms dislodging and flooding my body with prickly fast anxiety.

The first time you feel how alone you are in the Universe is always at sunset. The changing sky intensifies your emotions as you feel life's ephemerality. Nature is always trying to teach us to let go. Why was it so easy for guys to let me go? I wish I had that gift, but instead, I felt a psychic bond after I merged with someone sexually that always turned to loss.

The cloud squiggles in the orange sky looked like fire-cracker smoke. I tried to take a picture on my phone, but it's hard to capture the fleeting energy of life. A picture of sunset is never the same as actually being there. It doesn't capture your emotion, or the gradual shimmer of change. I felt how much was beyond my control as traffic, the ocean, and the sky moved around me.

I dreamt that a relationship would be the antidote for my purposelessness. Other people give you a destination. You can land in them. Just being in conversation and touching, life is full. But alone, you are adrift to find meaning on your own. Why was it so hard to find somebody who wanted to fall into each other? Maybe I didn't talk enough, hadn't made a good impression? I racked my brain for answers about why it didn't work out so I could improve in the future.

The Sun sank behind the sea. The Earth was moving, but where to? Maybe I had to accept there was no destination. It was dusk now and the air was purple. Everything that had been solid and golden earlier was now uncertain. The change from day to night triggers an inner shift. As the seen world fades, emotions get louder.

Now the squiggle clouds turned orange. Cheetos in a navy sky. I reached out to grab them just as they faded, ungraspable. The day was over. I stood there in shock. I had still been hoping he'd pull up. Damn, this was aloneness. It felt like a magnet was pushing my stomach away. Maybe this is how realizing you are pregnant feels—when something deep inside you has changed. This was the feeling of emptiness I'd been avoiding.

Venus glowed in the sky. The Goddess of Love, in her evening star phase. Are gods real or just stories to blame our pain on? I had felt Love, but also its absence. Or maybe I hadn't felt real Love yet? I had peak moments and then this emptiness would always return, the space of joy departed. I wanted to heal this, but the more I touched the feeling, the worse the pain of aloneness got, pulling me in. I got back in the car, its lights dimmed on calmly as I opened the door. I checked Schlong again. Was this thing on? Was my phone broken? Was the Universe broken? How could you merge so deeply with someone and then never want to talk to them again?

I started the car. I thought of Thelma and Louise-ing it off the cliff, but it seemed too soon. There was still so much I wanted to understand. And write about. I sat in my car breathing into my tingly body. It was anxiety and aliveness. It was the other side of merging, un-fucking, crash landing back into yourself.

The car was idling and the odometers waited peacefully. Aloneness was having so much to share but no one to share it with. I thought about looking for him at the fish restaurant, but I felt too activated to interact with any humans. I was in the neighborhood of Greta Garbo and Cher, near their castles of success. I was so close to LA wealth and happiness, but completely outside it, alone on this cliff. I opened the car door and screamed "FUUHHCKK." The ocean absorbed it like pee, too small to make any difference. I slammed on the horn and realized, like everything else in my life, it didn't work.

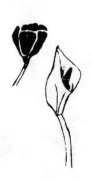

10

Good Vibrations

A skylight cast a glow over the shelves of serums, herbs, cacti and us glowing shop workers. It was always cold in the shop, to preserve the juices and the customers alike from the LA heat. After two months, I was finding my stride with the daily tasks of the job: restocking, making smoothies, placing the bottles just so, ringing up sales on the iPad. The job was a blend of barista, retail, herbalist, and dinner party host. Small talk is an overlooked skill in the service industry. It's hard to do well and it gives so much to the world. Service workers who interact with kindness can save your life. Have you ever had a waitress call you "honey" when you were feeling unloved, and started crying, and then she brought you free blueberry pancakes? More than just tasks, there's a maintaining of humanity and friendliness you uphold as a good retail clerk. I say "have a good day" to hundreds of customers a day, and I honestly mean it.

My favorite product at the shop was Spirit Dust, the euphoric, anti-anxiety herb blend. It made me feel lighter and less mental. The main ingredient is Reishi, the Chinese herb that soothes the heart and opens the psychic senses. Mimosa bark has since been removed from the formula because it is psycho active in large amounts. I started testing the limits of how much Dust I could handle. I put it in my chai and felt sparkly, my eyelids heavier. I felt good but could I feel even better? I added it to a matcha, then stirred another teaspoon into a dash of California Sun. I felt ethereally peaceful all day and the shift flew by. The lady whose matcha is never hot enough didn't bug me, I just re-made it adding in the psychic intention that she no longer find fault with everything. When I went to count my cash drawer at closing, my mind was so loose I kept losing the number I was on and had to keep starting over. I never went beyond one serving of Spirit Dust after that.

The Dust had a cult following among the regulars who also felt its not-so-subtle benefits. "Mommy needs her Spirit Dust," a woman said, clacking her nails on the counter as her kid practiced gymnastics next to the cacti. I could see why she needed it. As I delivered her Spirit Chai, her kid somersaulted into a shelf and shattered three jars of Pearl powder. I swept it up after they left and scattered it off the balcony behind the shop. I hoped the wind would carry the Pearl blessing to whoever needed its soothing luster.

My Juice Shop training had taught me that stress is the leading cause of disease and the effects of aging. The jars of herbs were blended to help different goals: beauty, focus, immunity, sleep. When customers asked, "is this stuff placebo?" I recommended they try Spirit Dust first, as it had the most palpable effect. The other herbs needed to build up over time. Some just liked the packaging, but once you felt the effects you were hooked. At one point we ran out of Spirit Dust due to its popularity. The mom came in everyday asking if it was back yet. I wanted to share some of our private stash with her, but the staff needed it to stay in a good mood, an unspoken part of our job.

"The scientologist is here!" I announced to my co-worker Lauren, who was misting herself with rose water. We hit the face testers to stay dewy throughout our shift. I don't know how we'd found out he was a scientologist, but that's how well we got to know the customers. They told us their ills and we recommended what to put in their smoothie and which jars they should take home. He was a nice guy and looked like a TV newscaster. "I'll take the Chocolate Force with ashwanguh." He always forgot a syllable but I didn't try to correct him. The herb was Ashwagandha from India, an adaptogen, a class of herbs being studied for their ability to balance the nervous system's stress responses. He slammed the $18 smoothie in one gulp and tossed the cup in the trash as he glided out.

There were three tip options on the screen when customers signed their credit card charge: 20%, 25% and 30%. Many people chose 30 and it changed my life. Do you know how good it feels to get a big tip? I think everyone should be required to work a service job for two weeks every couple of years, like jury duty, to put you in someone else's shoes. It's hard to serve people, remembering all the substitutions and special requests, staying calm when it's busy, and standing around when it's slow. No one is being nice to you at a service job for free. It's a trade of our energy for your energy. Say it with tips. Tipping is a way to redistribute wealth. It's a personal gesture of human-to-human appreciation. Thank you for being. Tipping isn't money lost, but a way to bless someone. I want to get rich just so I can be a big tipper.

"Do you know what time it is?" Lauren asks. She is half Elvira and half Farrah Fawcett, a witchy babe. "It's Matcha time." I love working with her because we can banter dad humor and puns all day. People groan in disapproval when they overhear us.

"Xoxo, Matcha Girl," I say.

"Matcha do about nothing."

"Is this too matcha or just right?" she asks. Re-applying bright coral lipstick. Smiling, her teeth covered in matcha.

"Have you ever snorted matcha?" I ask.

"Nah, I don't snort shit no more," she says seriously.

"I've been obsessed with The Beach Boys studio outtakes," I tell her as I unbox new Hawaiian face serums onto the retail shelves. Lauren and I are both music nerds and cross pollinate information. As I pick off drooping flowers from an arrangement I expand. "Their basslines are sick. Hypnotic. I always loved them for the Cali Sunshine vibes, but they are actually such good musicians."

She's packing a delivery order and tosses her black ponytail with a natural skunk streak in it. "Agreed. But you know all that sunshine is kind of a facade. You know how messed up Brian Wilson was? Their dad used to beat them if they didn't make hit songs, so the sunshine was coming from this twisted place." I paused in awe to process this news. I could see something in my story in The Beach Boys: Reaching for happiness as a cover up for pain.

On my lunch break, I get my headphones and walk down Sunset. The shop is so cold it always feels good to be in the Sun for my 30-minute lunch break. I can see straight down to the Hollywood Sign. I made up that you can wish on it, so every day on my break I make a wish. Today it is just the words "Rock and Roll." All of it. The music and the feeling. Rockers seemed able to handle all of life.

I usually go to Siete Mares and get fish tacos. Sitting at the table with drying lettuce and hot sauce spills, I read The

Beach Boys' history. I had no idea. Maybe everything has a shadow. Walking back to work I pass a man who looks shipwrecked on the cement. His pants are torn above his ankles. He's passed out and is literally roasting, sweating from the Sun. I am scared to wake him though, not knowing what his response might be. His Air Jordans are ripped, yellow foam oozing out the tongue. No one sees him from their cars. Will he just simmer until he gets naturally cremated? I am listening to "Good Vibrations" as I consider what to do. I have to get back to work on time, so look to the Hollywood Sign and pray he gets some help. If people were half as interested in helping others as they are in their own health and beauty, we could get a lot done.

Coming into the shop from Sunset is always a relief. The line has built up and I greet some regulars as I put on my apron and clock back in. There's a vibration of care and luxury that brings meaning to people's lives in the shop, and I get to be a source of education and encouragement for people's wellbeing. Healing spaces bolster your spirits with the good parts of life. And the shop is good for me. The clear structure of my days at work was teaching me to find joy in the simple tasks of daily life. I restocked, rearranged, took orders and cleaned up with care and integrity. The only part I dreaded was washing the wellness shot cups. I didn't mind the blenders or measuring spoons, but these were gross. After people drank from them, we put them in a bucket of sanitizing solution. By the end of the shift, there were 30 cups and the water had turned brown and smelled sharply of oregano,, turmeric and people's mixed saliva. I picked it up and took it to the back dutifully. If only I could do as good a job for myself as I did when employed by someone else.

Dara was subletting an apartment near the Juice Shop and she invited me over for a lunch meeting. She looked like a brown fairy wearing a black tube top with arm bands attached. She always made everything she wore exponentially cooler.

"Lunch is ready, are you hungry?"

She had told me it was her interior designer friend's apartment and I had to see it. She pointed out things as we walked through the living room. Every surface was painted in a mural—geometric designs or faux architectural fixtures, in brown, maroon and gold. It was cool, but what was it? Moroccan or Mediterranean? Old Hollywood? I couldn't quite place the influence, maybe it was made up. It felt like we were inside a dreamy cartoon. She led me to the kitchen.

We sat down to the macro-bowls she had prepared. Dara's beauty seeps into everything she does and I was looking forward to imbibing her vibe through this gorgeous meal of greens, black rice and edible flowers.

"Bless," she said, putting her hands together in prayer. I

did the same. Silently we sank in for a few breaths. "Grateful for you," I said. "Grateful to you," she replied, opening her sparkly eyes.

"So what's your business idea?" I asked, taking my first bite.

"We are going to be the next Ram Dasses," she said, taking a bite of spinach into her frosted blue lips.

"Wow, how do these mushrooms taste like bacon?"

"Umami powder, fried in coconut oil baby," she said, and continued the business pitch.

"There are so many people online who are hungry for who we are. There are casting people looking for us. We just need to put out the vision for them to hook into."

"But I feel like I am too complicated for a world that wants to know what you are in a word, or a sentence," I said.

"Lukey, you are living a liberated vibration. You are freeing up from the confines of who or what you should be. People need to hear that. We just need a video person, a makeup and hair person, and some PR."

Our conversations were mental sex. We free-associated, encouraging and fertilizing each other's new ideas. I thought we could do a podcast, but would our conversations lose their spontaneity and become self-conscious when we were recording them?

"Let's just do a pilot to see where it goes. We hang out, like we normally do, but film it. Let me take a quick shower and we can set it up on the veranda. Will you make us a tonic? You can use anything in the kitchen."

I put the kettle on and went to look at the books in the hallway. They were thick and leather bound with gold embossed letters. I pulled one out and realized they were glued together. They were just props. I looked at the other shelves, some were real books, but had been chosen because they matched the dark spine and gold letter style. The surrealness made me second-guess if I'd slipped out of reality? It made me think of that essential theme of LA: substance versus appearance. In a magazine or movie this would have looked totally cool, but actually being inside it was weird and fake.

By the time Dara came out of the shower it was time for me to go back to work.

"You wanna do it quick? I have to go in like fifteen."

"Oh no! I still have to do my hair."

"I'm sure Ram Dass wouldn't care if you had wet hair," I said.

"Ya, but I want people to see you can have beauty and soul," she said, stroking on Egyptian style wet eyeliner.

"Where the tonics at?"

I jumped up to check on the kettle that had been boiling for a while. I poured hot water into the blender and started adding each of the expensive superfoods Dara had. A spoon of "Nine Immortals" mushroom blend, a full squeeze of "Blue Lotus Drops." A smidge of crimson paste called "Yoni Power." And the most expensive of all, a "Pineal Gland Decalcifier," which was made of ground up meteorites. I blended it up and poured the frothy, steaming elixir into two mugs and took it to the bathroom.

"Thanks fwiend," she said in her baby voice that always made me chuckle. I sat on the edge of the tub while she flat-ironed her hair. Two painted vases of flowers framed the real mirror.

"Do you think some of the celebrities from Venus Juice want to be on our show?"

The tonic was too hot and I spit it back into the mug. "No dude, I don't know them like that. I'm just a worker there. Plus, I don't want to do a reality TV show, as much as I love you! I like herbs and spirituality but I don't want to be famous for that. I don't want to be boxed into liking something and being an expert. I just want to be. Wasn't Ram Dass all about being nobody?"

She picked up her tonic and rolled her eyes as she took a sip. I secretly hoped we would do something together because part of me did want to be somebody. Different parts of me wanted conflicting things.

A few weeks later, Dara had moved on to another career idea. She had started dating the owner of a night club and they would stop at the shop to get coffee and snacks to last them until close at 2am. "Lukey, I'm going to be a celebrity death doula. I am going to do the training next month. Celebrities are an

untapped niche, they need help dying just like everyone else."
She looked like a sexy vampire in a black mesh coat and red velvet choker.

"That is so insane it might just work. I think you'd be a beautiful person to guide people to cross over," I said.

"Is the Sex Dust vegan?" her boyfriend asked.

"Ya, everything here is vegan. Except pearl. And honey."

"Okay, sweet, let me get a double Sex Brain latte."

I gave a double thumbs up and went to make it.

"You want anything else babe?" he asked her. His beard was brindled with brown, red and white hair. His hair in a messy bun. He had started paying for everything in Dara's life in exchange for her quitting sex work. After I made his latte, they drove off in his red Tesla and I got to taking the trash out.

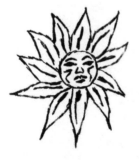

11

Opal Teardrop

After work one night in September my coworker invited me to a party on a patio in Echo Park. I had been in LA for four months and was meeting new friends, enjoying my job, and learning the roads in my new car. The patio glowed with Christmas lights and people chatted, drinking kombucha and smoking cigarettes. Patios in LA are open year-round, they always seem to have a faded canvas umbrella and cacti. The cool desert nights were a relief from the hot fall days.

Curiosity over the guy in the bedazzled cap sitting in the group next to me built up. He had glassy Chihuahua eyes and long blonde hair. His hands and body were strong but also feminine. The hat gave him a 2000s Britney Spears vibe, but his clothes made him look like a carpenter. Someone finally introduced us and I asked him about his hat. He'd gotten it at a truck stop near Joshua Tree. We talked about how surreal that area is. Turns out he lived nearby and wanted to show us his house. Conveniently, I was the only one who wanted to go, so I would have him all to myself.

We walked to my car and when I opened the car door the alarm went off, making dogs start barking and breaking the silence of what had been a peaceful Thursday night. I was still discovering problems with the Lexus I'd bought off Craigslist. I knew once I started the car the alarm would stop, but I still hadn't figured out what kept triggering it. I turned the gold plated "L" key in the ignition and the alarm stopped and the oldies came on the radio. We drove off.

How anyone could get into my destroyed Lexus and not comment on it was surprising. It's noteworthy whether you think it's funny or tragic. Maybe it just seemed like a Camry to him, which it basically was, but with a sleek wood console and interior lights that dimmed slowly on and off. The fact that he didn't appreciate this car was a bit of a red flag.

But now that we were alone he lost his shyness. "Who are you?! Where did you come from?!" he asked in excitement. I smiled, but froze, not wanting to mess this up like I had with the other guys. I couldn't think of anything to say, so just smiled awkwardly. "That's me," he said pointing to a brown shingled cabin on a platform off the side of the hill.

"The house was built by a lesbian couple in the 1970s," he said as we walked in. It looked like a set for a 70s gay porn film. A California flag hung over the stone fireplace. A striped serape covered his couch.

AL – wishing you DEC '21
a very happy
birthday – may this
year be brimming with
juicy abundance,
creativity + nourished
spirit. This book
really resonated w/
me. I hope you like it.

♡ ya – B

"Let's sit outside, it's such a nice night," he said.

He led me to his patio, which was decorated with Christmas lights, an old canvas umbrella, and octopus-like agave plants.

"So, what do you do?" he asked, stretching back in his chair.

"Besides the Juice Shop, I've been working on music."

"Oh ya? I love music. What kind of music do you play?"

"I play guitar and sing. Still finding the sound."

"You should sing me something," he said.

One of my favorite Fleetwood Mac songs was playing from inside the house, so I sang along: *Rock on gold dust woman, take your silver spoon and dig your grave.*

As I sang, I realized my singing voice was just a louder version of my speaking voice, so I tried harder. *Lousy lovers, pick their prey but they never cry out loud*, I harmonized, not holding back. *Did she make you cry? Make you break down? Shatter your illusions of Love? And is it over now, do you know how? Pick up the pieces and go home.* Now I felt warmed up and ended with a low croon: *Pick up the pieces and go hohhmmme.*

"Wow you're good," he said, a beat after I finished.

"Thanks. What do you do?" I asked.

"Trying to paint. But mostly fixing up the house."

"Woah, with tools?" He nodded. "Hot," I said.

He got up and reached out his hand and led me inside to sit on the sheepskin in the living room. We eye gazed for a few seconds. His eyes were like a shiny black puppy's, with a skittishness. I felt his hand on my cheek and as he tilted his head to kiss me I closed my eyes. Lip skin is so perceptive. There's silent communication that happens between lip skin when you kiss. The Cher song "It's in His Kiss" is right, you can tell so much about someone by the rhythm and quality of their kiss.

His kiss was thoughtful and gentle. He slid his sparkly hat off and I ran my hand through his hair. He eased us to lay down. We were getting to know each other silently, through sensations. Making out is healing in its best moments, like an emotional massage. I felt my nervous system relaxing. I passed the test, we were merging.

He pulled my shirt off and I felt the silky fur under me. My mind was lost in the sureness of his tongue and hands. "Take this off," I said, tugging his t-shirt up. The contours of his muscles shadowed in the dim light. Something shifted and it got more primal. We started rolling around and it went into this wrestling mating ritual. Caveman chemicals were being emitted as we panted and sloppily kissed. I paused and caught his eyes. He was taken off guard. He seemed scared, unsure what to do. I smiled, giving him a sparkle that showed how much I wanted this to be our life. A smile that showed him how much I have to give.

He smiled back and asked, "what are you smiling at?"

"How hot you are," I replied.

"No, you are," he said.

I could see the imprint of his hard-on in his jeans and reached for his jeans button. "You should take these off."

"I really want to. But I want to save that for later," he said.

We did everything you can do with clothes on and then hugged in silence. Outside the dark window I could see the distant car lights moving on the freeway. The outside world seemed so calm in this warm and cozy moment with him. Being with someone always felt like being caught, no longer free-falling into the abyss. "Let's do this again soon," he said. I drove home with a peaceful afterglow.

I woke up the next day with Rihanna in my head. My spontaneous hook-up had rejuvenated me and I was excited to get to know him more. I sent him the song "Diamonds" with lots of emojis, but he didn't reply.

He finally texted that afternoon, while I was sitting at the patio table.

Thanks for coming over. I don't want to hang again.

My cells scattered in shock and disappointment. I didn't know how to deal with all the feelings, so I just laid in the Sun, paralyzed. Are all queer people wounded in intimacy, I wondered? Because we experienced shame and rejection growing up, do we feel un-worthy of Love? Sex gives you a moment of intimacy, but why couldn't we go deeper? I couldn't believe the dude couldn't give a little more vulnerable explanation about why he didn't want to hang out again.

That afternoon, when I finally had enough energy to take a shower, I realized I'd lost my opal teardrop earring. I hadn't taken it off since I bought it two years ago in New Mexico, and it reminded me of home. My mind went back to his hands grabbing my hair and neck last night. I felt robbed.

I texted him back: "Did my earring fall off on the sheepskin?"

The animated ellipsis showed that he was typing.

... "Ya it's here. Come by and get it whenever."

... "Now?"

... "Sure."

It was dark when I got there and I parked in the same spot I had the night before, but now my first date anxiety was replaced by the hurt of rejection. The streetlight shined a cool fluorescent blue over his doorstep. As I knocked I felt a sadness I wasn't sure was mine or his. He cracked the door. There was no music on in his house. What was he doing in there? Was he alone? He looked just as hot, but there was an absence in his eyes, like he wasn't even seeing this scene.

"Here it is." He opened his hand with the teardrop in it. It was like seeing an organ out of your body. I plucked it up, but the moment I touched it I knew I couldn't put it back on. I swallowed and tried to compose all my emotions into a non-confrontational question, but I just said it plain: "Why don't you want to hang out again?"

His face was half-shadowed by the cracked door. He didn't want to come out and he didn't want me to come in. "There are things about me you don't know. There are things about me no one knows. I'm sorry I just can't."

We locked eyes for a split second of silence, then he closed the door and I heard it lock.

I stood in the blue light, listening to the freeway, waiting for him to open the door again, because this was not finished. This hadn't even begun. The blue flowers on the bush by his door had dew drops on their petals. Maybe they were crying. How can you show someone so much in a moment and then take it back? I stood there because I wasn't ready to face the anxious night of investigating what I'd done wrong. A breeze reminded me that I'd been holding my breath since he closed the door. I crawled through my open car window so I wouldn't set off the alarm.

Waking up the next morning my sadness had a tinge of fire to heal my relationship disappointments once and for all. When something happens three times it is a clear message the Universe is trying to get your attention. Pablo had disappointed me. Ballet Surfer had ghosted me. Maybe it wasn't just bad luck, and I was playing a role in how things had played out. I decided to call on my healer Mike Kelly. His healing sessions are $300, so I only book one when it's a life-or-death situation.

Fortunately Mike could see me the next day and he's not afraid to hold space for difficult moments. That's why he's a good healer. He teaches a specific kind of breathwork, a rhythmic breathing meditation that gets energy and emotions moving. He guides people back to the Love of the Universe. I'd known him for five years and he has seen me in my darkest and brightest moments. A true healer can hold all parts of you. I aspired to be like Mike, one day helping people. But, for now, I still felt like his student, trying to get through my own stuff.

It was a sunny morning when I pulled up to Mike's Mediterranean villa in Montecito Heights. It has a balcony perfect for a production of Romeo & Juliet. I forgot my wallet in the car and set off the alarm again when I opened the door.

"Heard you were here from the alarm," Mike said as I approached the front door. We hugged and I stepped into his huge house. There were framed blue butterflies on the walls and an altar of shells and crystals on the fireplace mantle. Downstairs was an open floor plan room with a TV nook, a kitchen and dining room table, all looking out to the pool. He lived there with his wife and new baby. He had the type of purposeful career, Love relationship and home I hoped for.

"You're living the dream," I said.

"Yup, we're pretty blessed. You need the bathroom?"

We passed through the kitchen, which vibrated with aliveness from just being cleaned up after breakfast. Mike's cat Kitty meowed near her cat bowl, wanting seconds. That he named his cat Kitty tells you a lot about his directness as a person. Just call it what it is, kitty. Just call it what it is, old patterns of negative thinking. Just call it what it is, looking outside yourself for Love. His gift was in untangling the mess of emotions and helping you just call it out.

The healing room was down a hallway on the first floor, and had great daylight. A candle flickered on the altar with an array of teeth, claws, and carved animals laid on a grey rabbit pelt. A hanging prism cast a spray of rainbows on the wall. We sat in chairs facing each other and I felt happy to be back in his care. He wore a faded purple t-shirt and his cheeks were rosy from living in Southern California for over twenty years. His hair was graying, but he had the youthful glow of people who have tapped into the eternal. His voice maintained the drawl of his Kentucky roots.

"So I guess your honeymoon period with LA is coming to an end? There's always the first couple of months where you can forget your problems, but they always come back, no matter how far away you try to run. How long's it been Luke?" He took a piece of beef jerky from a sandwich bag near his essential oils and took a bite while I did the math in my head.

"A little over three months."

He chewed and looked at me like he was inspecting a repair that was going to be complicated. I sipped from the tall glass of water he'd gotten me.

"So who is this guy?"

"I guess I don't really know, that's the problem."

He shook his head yes. "And how did you meet?"

"At a party, friend of friends. He had an amazing house, we had an amazing night together, and then he didn't want to hang out again. And I know I shouldn't be feeling so vulnerable and hurt, that I have to be more careful with my heart, but it's so frustrating, and sad. I just wanna be with someone." I grabbed the conveniently placed box of Kleenex and dabbed the tears that were starting.

"Look, you're doing great. You've really come a long way, Luke, you know that. You're still right in there, you're still attracting these lessons for a reason—to mirror this uncertainty around Love. These guys are just showing you your own unsureness around your lovability. Do you think you're lovable?" He took another bite of beef jerky and chewed while I thought about it.

I looked out the window for the answer. The Sun lit up the dust in the air like gold glitter, and I could see my car parked happily outside. That is MY Lexus, I thought. Even if I am having another heartbreak, at least I have a car now and can afford an expensive healing session. I had come a long way. One of Mike's messages for me was always to out-create my hopelessness with Love. To look on the bright side rather than spiral into old feelings of distress. It was like the visioning I learned from Dana. I imagined myself leaning against my car wearing marquee shaped sunglasses, happy. "Ya, I guess I am lovable," I finally said.

A bird hit the window with a smack. We paused to see if it flew off, but it didn't. "Well I guess that's a confirmation from Spirit. You gotta be more careful with those closed windows," he said.

My body was getting tingly. Mike is an energy worker and just being around him can make you feel like you are going to sob or burst out laughing from emotions. Just by feeling seen and heard, my distress was lifting. His presence itself was healing. Mike was going easy. I already knew he was going to tell me to take responsibility and not blame others, to free myself from the inside.

"When you leap fast you have less time to see where you're gonna land," Mike said. That felt like a punch in the stomach, but ouch, it was true. I had blamed these guys for rejecting me, but maybe it was me who moved too fast and set the stage for my own disappointment.

"Do you want something fast or do you want something slow?"

I laughed, "Both."

He laughed, "Well, what do you want?"

"A loving partner."

"Okay, go on. You gotta create it. In your mind. You gotta draw it, paint it, envision it, feel it. That's how you manifest. You gotta out-create the negativity with Love. What type of shoes does he have? What type of car does he have? Maybe he has a truck, and cowboy boots, I could see that for you."

I laughed. Mike was always guiding me back to humor to get me out of my dark seriousness.

"I just want to be in Love."

"Do you love yourself?"

I paused and looked for the answer on the ceiling this time. "Sometimes."

He stood up and put his hand on the massage table, "Come on up."

My eyes covered by a silk eye pillow and my hands gripping a pair of ocean stones, I started the breath pattern. Since I had trained with him, I didn't need to be reminded of how to breathe. I went right into the rhythmic pattern that hyper-oxygenates the blood and takes you on a natural psychedelic journey. As I breathed, the sadness in my heart fluttered awake like embers stoked back to a flame. It was just under the surface, the rawness, the hurt, the disappointment. No romance ever worked out, what was wrong with me?

"Good breathing, I hope you like country," he said, keeping me from getting distracted by thought. "That was a joke," he said. And I laughed at the fact that he always has to point out his bad jokes. He played an angelic acoustic cover of "Wonderwall" by LeAnn Rimes. I sang along; *Maybe, you're gonna be the one that saves me.* Using my voice made me want to cry more, but I couldn't, I was too stiff, habitually gripping onto my mind to avoid my feelings. Mike intuitively picked up on my stuckness. "Come on Luke, breathe," he said, patting my belly and heart to quicken my breath pace. He brushed some essential oils on my throat. Having him there kept me present, and gave me strength to push through and feel it.

Before I met Mike my emotions were muddy and frozen. He would ask, "how does it make you feel?" and I'd say "I don't know."

Thoughts are safe, emotions can get wild. I wanted to experience Love, and that meant I had to face the backed-up shit clogging my emotional plumbing. Breathwork disrupts the familiar patterns of feeling and helps our subtle energy circulate. It gives a direct experience of the energy body, emotions, and intuition. Reclaiming our direct experience is the first step of owning who we really are. You have to look into the dark pools and own it in order to forgive it. It helps to have someone to hold your hand, and help push you beyond your comfort zone.

In the healing room Cat Stevens "Wild World" came on. I breathed steadily into my belly and heart, and exhaled angrily. I hated this. My body felt like heavy metal. I hated that I was paying money to heal from a stupid one night stand. I was mad at the Universe for doing this to me, why couldn't I just find someone? I started to cry, gasping.

"And you're still lovable," Mike's voice chimed in, "Go ahead and say, 'I'm lovable.'"

"I'm," gasp, "lovable."

"I'm a catch."

I squirmed from full body shivers. "I'm a," gasp, "catch."

"And I'm enough."

The pain dissolved away. My body got heavy, and my voice deepened three octaves: "I'm enough."

"Good. This is probably a good place to shift into the normal breath," Mike said, burning a sage leaf to clear away what I'd released into the air. He changed the music to a sitar raga.

"So what do you want?"

I lay there, deeply clear now. "I want someone who's available for something deep."

"Are you deep?"

"Yup."

"What do you love about yourself?"

"My deep emotions."

"Good, think of 10 more things. I'm gonna go feed kitty."

Laying on the table I felt Love for the rainbow of emotions and moods I have inside. I felt peace beneath all the ups and downs. I had found my way back to a stable, neutral part of myself. This is where I wanted to live. I wanted to make this my set point, my home base. I knew that my path was learning to return back to this feeling of Love inside and around me. I sniffled and sat up. Sage smoke floated in the bright room. I was starving. I reached for the bag of jerky he had been working on and ate a piece.

12

The Diamond Earring

After I retrieved the opal earring, it felt too charged with disappointment to put back in. I needed a new earring. I visited Dream Collective, the jewelry store I had hoped a guy would one day buy me something from. But I was done trying to get things from guys. I was committed to becoming the lover I was seeking, and this gift to myself would commemorate this inner marriage.

Dream Collective is more than a shop, it's a mood brought to life. There are birds of paradise in violet vases, clean lines of modern furniture upholstered in knotty cream linen, a stained-glass window of a huge eye. You pass through the scented bath and home accessories to the jewelry part of the shop in the back. The glass case has delicate gold rings with the outline of an eye with a single ruby as the pupil. Or a gold snake ring with rainbow sapphires around the tail and a diamond as its eye.

As my own boyfriend, I couldn't afford everything I

wanted, but I could swing an earring. "Can I see that triangle diamond stud?" I asked the clerk with swoop bangs. She unlocked the case and pulled it out for me. "Can you buy just one stud, or do I have to buy both?"

"You can just buy one. What's the price for just one stud?" she asked the owner through a little window to the back office. I loved hearing the word "stud" thrown around. A single stud, I'd found my stud, this was the stud for me.

"Do you have any blood diamonds here?" I asked.

Shocked, the clerk replied, "absolutely not. You would get a paper with the diamond verifying that it was consciously mined." This quelled my conflicting desires for luxury and doing no harm.

I had worked with crystals but never diamond before. In Indian astrology, gems are used to balance planetary energies. Diamond represents Venus. I held the earring by the post and studied the diamond in the light—it was silver, still some charcoal in its carbon. Imperfect but sparkly, just like me. A spell was forming itself in my mind. I could use the earring as a reminder to love myself and life, even when it got hard. I liked the symbolism that diamonds are created through long periods of compression into their strong, durable beauty.

"I'll take it."

I opted for a screw back rather than a rubber stopper that could be dislodged again while making out. The idea of having a diamond bolted to my ear fit my intention for the spell, which was to always react with Love, no matter what.

I waited until Friday to cast the spell. Friday, the day of Venus, had become a holy day for me, because I am a Libra, ruled by the planet of Love. Each day is like a movie directed by a different planet, giving each day its different vibe. There's an exhale and excitement in the air on Friday, as people finish the work week and get liberated to pleasure and play. I had finally found a rhythm in LA. I worked the weekend at the Juice Shop and had started teaching yoga Saturdays and breathwork Sundays, so Friday was my Monday. It was important to fill up my cup, to kick it off in high spirits.

My Friday ritual was sound tracked by my favorite DJ's weekly radio show, "Things of Life," which I listened to on headphones from 10am-noon. Everybody, the queer gym, had opened nearby, and I drove over Mount Washington to Frogtown. I would wear a choker necklace and pink Vans, and do the row machine to get my blood pumping, not feeling self-conscious because of Everybody's inclusive mission statement and community. Exercise made me feel grounded, it burned off my nerves. I had never learned how good working out makes you feel because I had never been a jock. There were orange trees on the gym's patio, and while I struggled to bench-press, psychedelic house music blasting in my ears, I smelled the orange blossoms: this is paradise, I thought. After working out, my endorphins were high, my appetite up, I headed home to cook and get ready to cast the spell while listening to the second hour of my pump-up radio show.

The sky that morning was bright blue. My roommates were already at work, so I could get witchy. I got the tiny box the earring came in and set it on the patio concrete. I picked up a twig and used it as a wand to cast a sacred circle, turning to the four directions and asking the land to help me. Then I turned the hose on to wash the diamond. Water gushed out like liquid silver. As I poured water over the earring in my palm, I asked it to release any old energy, so it could fully hold my prayer. Water spilled on my feet, and I decided to just shower out there with the hose. I took my clothes off and shivered as cold water dripped from my hair down my back. It's always adds potency when you do magic naked.

I held the earring to the Sun. I asked the Goddess Venus to help my heart heal, and to enter the diamond and gold. Then I pressed it to my heart and filled the diamond with my own heart, palms crossed over it, still dripping, in silence. May I learn to bring this Love into every interaction and respond with Love to whatever happens. I slipped the gold rod in and screwed the earring backer on. Then I spun counterclockwise a few times to close the circle.

I was feeling exuberant as I made lunch, put on my white

work clothes and headed out. I believe spells work to remind us that life is flexible and full of possibilities. Maybe magic is more for influencing ourselves than for influencing the out- side world, but who knows? "That's how magic works, by magic," Starhawk once said at a workshop I took.

The ritual and the diamond itself gave me a sensual memo- ry and a physical touchstone to remind me of the change I was making inside. My life already felt more beautiful and hopeful.

Sometimes a spell works by bringing something up to the sur- face to be released. A week later I woke up sweating with a fever. I fumbled to the bathroom. My stomach hurt, I didn't know if I was going to vomit or have diarrhea. It was the latter. I lay in bed watching the Sun rise out the patio doors. It turned into a hot day and I shivered and sweated in bed. I called in sick to work and hobbled back to the bathroom. I imagined the months of built-up vitamins and minerals from all that juice being wasted. My micro-biome I had nourished with fer- mented foods was being obliterated. But, the strength of the fever was a good sign that my immune system was strong and working to defend itself.

The next day my manager at the Juice Shop urged me to go to the hospital. Not because she thought I was lying, but because she was genuinely concerned after hearing me over the phone. None of my friends were available to take me, so I held the fence as I went down the stairs to my Lexus. I felt like I was floating in my car to Pasadena and definitely should not have been driving. At the emergency room I kept sliding out of the chair, my body was so weak.

I was led to a private hospital room with shiny linoleum flooring and they had me change into a hospital gown. It was soft cotton but I was freezing. "It will be good for you to be cold to cool the fever," they said. I was pretty sure you wanted to help the body burn out the toxins, but I shelved my holistic health knowledge and put my trust in the allopathic ways. I had a fever of 105 but they said it was just dehydration. This was curious because I drank so much juice? But, it had been really hot during the days. They gave me an IV of intravenous fluids. I laughed thinking of IVs full of green juice. I had passed from the pain part into a sort of zen hilariousness.

Having not eaten or slept in days I felt lucid. I laid in the silent hospital room and let go. I thought of Ram Dass, after having his stroke, his body bony, but eyes wet with inner peace. I meditated and felt connected to him. Maybe this was it. There was no holding on. If I died, would the guys who had betrayed me find out? *There are more fish in the sea*, Ram Dass's energy whispered to my intuition. Different male nurses checked on me hourly. I realized their care was the thing making me feel better, not necessarily whatever was in the IV.

The doctor, who looked like Santa, informed me it was

just a virus and to take Advil for the pain, rest and hydrate. I was discharged and headed to Walgreen's to get the Advil. Turning into the parking lot I accidentally rear-ended the car in front of me when they abruptly stopped. The driver got out. "Why the fuck did you hit my car?!" she screamed as I rolled down the window. I couldn't talk to the angry driver. I was shivering and holding back laughter. Sometimes you laugh as a weird response to stress. We both had insurance so I knew it would be okay. Shit happens. I should have asked her for a ride home. Usually I would have hated this day, being sick, the fender bender, making someone mad. But today I felt anchored in a deeper layer of Love and compassion for it all. Holy shit, the spell was working. I pulled down the rear-view mirror and looked at my diamond earring glinting in the Sun.

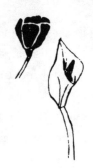

13
Natural Healing

In a lull at work I researched hikes, and decided to go once I got off the morning shift. Since I passed the six-month mark and got promoted to assistant manager, the shop started feeling like a normal job. The initial learning curve and uphill climb had been realized. Now the high-maintenance customers and their dietary restrictions annoyed me. I was tired of talking up the benefits of natural beauty products and balancing herbs. I wanted to be in Nature and get the direct experience. Maybe what was making us imbalanced was our total disconnection from Nature and obsession with work? The shop was empty and I looked out to the endless passing cars. Everything in America was enclosed in glass, air conditioned, and divided up into single portions. Everybody was working to get theirs. I wanted to take all the herb jars on the hike and liberate them back to the land. I wanted to pour myself out of the jar of who I thought I was or should be.

I got stuck in traffic on my way to the mountains and was

disturbed by how few cars were in the carpool lane. All of us were alone in our own cars. Finally we started flowing and I could see the San Gabriel Mountains in their full glory. If you can withstand the frustrating slow downs, the roads will lead to pristine places. The thought cut through my crankiness and I snapped back into faith that synchronicity was still guiding me.

I had started working five days a week at the Juice Shop since I'd been promoted to Assistant Manager. I had been proud of the achievement and pay raise, but now I was feeling drained and lost. I had been too exhausted to work on music or promote myself as a healer online. Why was I giving so much time and energy to this job that wasn't my life purpose? This was a familiar struggle I'd had at other jobs. Doing something just for the money always feels soul sucking. The new American dream is making money from your passion. I was tired of serving rich creatives. I wanted to be a rich creative. I wanted to get paid to be myself. I parked and breathed the higher elevation air. Nature is a relief because you don't have to be anybody or anything. I saw footprints in the dirt, someone had been hiking barefoot. We all need breaks from human society.

I followed the pale dirt trail that zig-zagged down the side of a mountain. White sage bushes burst with their sacred, purifying leaves. I was glad no one had picked it to bundle and sell. I sent the sage protection prayers as I passed and stroked it. The plant has been over-harvested in our struggle to rid the world of negative energy. I don't ever use the words "negative energy," though. For me, the problem is ego, disconnection from the heart. I can detect when I'm trapped in my head, my sense of self struggling to assert itself, to make sense, that's when I go to nature to reset.

Nature is the healer's healer. As I hiked, the bay laurel smell was potent, like mint soaked in whiskey. I wondered if I could make a cologne from it and sell it? I caught myself again in the constant search for how to make money off something. Why wasn't it enough just to exist? I wanted to learn to value things in their natural form, when they haven't been packaged and promoted. I snorted in the bay laurel and brush smells to re-wire myself back to Nature.

The guidebook said there was a stream in the canyon. I could discern the distant sound, and got quiet to listen. I could notice the difference without my noisy intellect. I walked the rest of the way down in an observant, walking meditation. The plants were more lush down by the creek, a happy trail, guiding me to the source of life.

A flat meditation rock on the side of the creek beckoned me. I sat down crossed-legged and closed my eyes. The constant gurgling sound guided my meditation. As thoughts fought for my attention the river sound kept bringing me back to just sitting. I blinked my eyes open and took in the lush creek bed around me. The Sun was glowing through the pine and laurel trees. I kept practicing letting my worries go, feeling the breeze on my t-shirt. As I let myself be influenced by the vibration of Nature, it tuned me like a guitar, out of the ego chatter. I didn't have to hold on so hard, I could be drawn like the creek, finding its way to the ocean. The thought sent me into quiet stillness, feeling the inter-relatedness of things.

At the end of my meditation I asked what my life's purpose was. The feeling in my heart made me laugh. Like my soul was tickling me from inside my heart. *Bringing new energy to Earth* were the words that had come along with the feeling. I realized, sitting there, that I got to do everything I loved at the Juice Shop—talk to people, make smoothies and tonics, listen to music, counsel people, stare out the window. I could feel God laughing at me. When would I learn to trust the flow of life? I felt ready to go back and enjoy my life, armed with this new understanding and reconnection to my purpose and my essence. It didn't matter where I was, I was going to keep being myself and grow this energy that made me feel happy.

I stood up, sent Reiki to the water and thanked it for healing me. For holding space for me to let go and clarify my mind. I had never felt Nature so alive, and wondered if it was the herbs in my system from the Juice Shop that had built up and bridged my consciousness into the plant realm? Walking back, the bare earth felt so much softer than concrete. I took off my sneakers and walked barefoot. I felt in awe of the Sierra Anita Ridge plants, river and hills, as well as the juice and herbs in my system, their magical ability to realign us to the Earth. The biggest mystery is under our feet.

14

Art

It took thirty years for me to be a musician and not just dress like one, but I am finally in a band. We go to the rehearsal space a few days a week to chip away at the block of granite that is our musical potential.

The band is me and Dee. Dee got laid off and is living on unemployment, committed to making music her life. Her bones are foxlike and she has the serious face of a porcelain doll. She is never out of costume—today she is wearing a rhinestone studded beret, a purple velvet turtleneck and lace gloves. It is 87 degrees and sunny.

"Aren't you hot?"

"Yeah, but I don't wanna get skin cancer. Ever since I moved to LA I keep getting more freckles. Are you wearing sunscreen?"

"I probably should."

My arms have been red since I moved here. The tan hasn't settled in, it is just a perpetual burn. Especially the left arm that I hang out the window while I drive.

There is a parking spot waiting for us next to a six-foot-tall jade plant. LA is plant heaven. I imagine when potted plants get thrown out they inch their way West to start a new life. That's what Dee and I did, too. We met in Brooklyn, but moved to LA where we'd have more time and space to be creative, in a warmer climate.

The practice room is damp and if you accidentally touch the carpet it is wet like an animal's nose. We light incense right away to cover up the stench. The first hour of practice we plug in our gear, drink juice, and update each other on our relationship developments. Having a band is like therapy. It costs about as much, and gives you similar benefits.

I thought coming to LA would inspire my sound. I wanted to catch the creative virus The Beach Boys had and write timeless pop melodies. I would be happy and make happy music. It's been the opposite. Our sound is chaos. Danielle's bass amp is blown out and shakes the room like thunder. My electric guitar notes screech like high pitched questions. We had both been betrayed by guys we'd met online and our thrashing was a cathartic outlet. There's how you think your art will be, and how it actually turns out.

Playing rock is narcotic. When you get into a jam and start improvising, you get high off the immediacy of your fingers, mind and sound. But sometimes you can't find it, you suck and wonder why you are even trying. You get hungry, thirsty, tired. I want to leave and go to the health food store for a kombucha. But we already have kombucha here. I've learned to prepare for this impulse by bringing a bag of snacks to every rehearsal. A bite of chocolate can quell that nagging ego critic voice to help you take that first step.

The jams last from 8 to 20 minutes and we take a break in between. We pop some more chocolate and do a dance break to our favorite song, "Believe" by Cher. It cheers us up that Cher believes there can be another life after Love. Then we jam again. No matter how much dance music we listen to, though, it never comes out in our sound. Our sound is muddy and intense. We have to play really loud to overpower the Mariachi music and traffic reports the broken PA system picks up. I wonder if our music isn't like a radio, and we are the receivers picking up on the Earth's climate crisis and painful histories. On the best days we lose track of time. The next renter bangs on the door and we quickly pack our gear and bag of snacks. Afterwards we're toast. Our chakras wide open and ears ringing, we re-emerge with our senses purified. We go back to the Lexus to find it is covered in purple flowers from the blooming jacaranda tree we parked under.

We always take a walk in Echo Park after playing music to come down. My body feels stronger and confident, tiger-like.

The park is an oasis: blooming lily pads, palm trees and a geyser fountain in the middle of the man-made lake. You completely forget the freeway is right there until you wash your face later and realize how much pollution you were in. Echo Park has the spontaneity I missed from New York. Everybody goes there—joggers, grandmas and kids on bikes. A woman records a fitness routine with her tripod oriented away from the cops telling park residents to move their tents.

I thought of a nice way to say what I wanted to say, but then I just said it: "I wish our music wasn't coming out so dark. I mean intense. It feels good, but it's not what I expected."

Dee paused, palm trees reflected in her sunglasses. "It is intense. I think there's a place for deep music, though. People fear emotions and try to make things more simple and palatable. I think we are releasing emotion through our music and we should go with it." Dee's commitment to art is pure and fearless.

There was a rainbow in the spray of the fountain. We paused to admire it. The prism came and went as the water got blown in the breeze. I thought of Virginia Woolf's essay "Moments of Being," how she translated living into words—steam curling from the soup pot. I wanted to capture the wonder, the vulnerability and mystery I felt. We all perceive life differently, like unique radios and cameras. And everything has been created. The park was someone's idea, just as the highway was someone's idea. Nature is God's art. The geyser kept spewing and the rainbow shimmered. We stood there in silence.

In that moment, I thought maybe I could just use words rather than trying to learn music. I loved art so much, and had tried for so long, but kept failing to create anything that resembled what I felt. The technical side of music was a stumbling block. Maybe I could use the language I already knew?

I'd struggled figuring out how to make art for years. In a healing session with Mike Kelly he said, "Don't worry about writing one good song, write 100 bad songs." Because I had such high expectations for the success of our band, I was constipated to actually create. "It's a billboard for your entire life," Mike said, "the fear it won't be perfect paralyzes you from actually doing it." Mike says creativity is the shortcut to healing, and encourages people to express their blocks through art to heal.

The band started good, but I quickly hit the same hollowness, and wanted to give up. I hated my voice. I couldn't make any good lyrics. And I wasn't that great at rhythm. In the practice space I could see the pattern in real time: this sucks, you suck, too corny, not original enough. I wanted it to be perfect right away, meaning I censored it before it even came out. But what is perfect? Dee wasn't mad about my impotence, she held a space for me to come through this birth canal. Collaboration is about enabling each other's creativity. The chaos WAS the sound. It was something. By embracing our raw sound I started to embrace whatever came through me artistically.

That summer art started infusing my life in a way I'd always dreamt of. Perceiving the moment and translating it into words gave my mind something to do other than spiral in existential confusion. I wrote in the morning and on my lunch break. Engaging artistically with life finally gave it meaning. I could write about it no matter what happened, it was all material to convey. Funny, when I let go of obsessing over how successful our band was going to be, we finally started writing songs.

We recorded our demo on the winter solstice, the last day we'd ever be in the rehearsal space. Even recording our songs I felt the same doubts, but we powered through. I wanted to feel what it's like to bring something into form. I had always given up on my art projects before. I loved the songs. They captured the tangle of beauty and pain we felt. Even if it wasn't "good," it was alchemy, we had turned our pain into art. I sang another take:

Petal by petal, opening to everything. I am a rose, don't need no one but myself. Bloom for myself. Make perfume when I wanna. The rose never reaches, the rose attracts her seekers.

Nobody listened to our songs when we released them, though. Or they did and didn't have anything nice to say about them.

We went to dinner at El Compadre a week later. I got enchiladas and Dee got a taco and another basket of free chips. "I guess nobody liked our jams," I said.

"It's not about who listens, but the experience. Besides, I just have fun making music with you, Luke." That took the edge off my feelings of failure. We watched as the waiter passed us with two blue flaming margaritas on a tray. Maybe the band had been a success just because we existed.

"Our band is so underground, only we know about it," I said. Dee laughed and dipped a chip into salsa with her lace gloves on.

I felt the bubble we lived in as friends, a delicate rainbow oil slick orb that we floated through the world in. It was better than fame to have one person who gets you. Just because you're not famous, doesn't mean you're not special.

15
The Party

On New Year's Eve, I invited the Dolphin Pod to watch *The Matrix* at the mansion I was housesitting. Someone had named our group text "Dolphin Pod" and it stuck as the name for our friend group. We were all playful and intuitive, like dolphins. Ruby made herbed popcorn and I had the refrigerator filled with juice bottles. Dee reclined on her side with mirrored sunglasses she'd worn for the occasion. "Be careful with that strawberry milk," I told her. I was watching over Mike Kelly's house while he taught a healing retreat, and I didn't want to spill on his all-white living room.

We'd all memorized lines from the movie and had started dressing in Matrix style cyber clothes. The pool glowed green outside as we turned the lights out and started the movie.

"Can we start a Matrix Church? Also, I need a black pleather jumpsuit," Dara said as her new muse Trinity backflipped off a wall. The movie was an oracle for the matrix we would face that year.

During my break at the Juice Shop a few weeks later, I checked my phone to find the Dolphin Pod group chat in a fight. Usually we shared YouTube music videos, invitations to gatherings or just expressed our gratitude for life and each other, so it was shocking that a fight had broken out. The texts kept arriving as I tried to catch up. The fight was about racism.

"You're the racist. Don't you think you are reinforcing dividing people by color?" Calvin wrote. Everyone was reacting in their own ways.

Dara: "If this friend group isn't racist then why am I the only person of color here?"

Calvin: "I would like to be considered a person of color too, I am Mexican."

Dara: "You're not dark enough, let me know when you have some black friends."

I wanted to come in with something diplomatic and pacifying. "Can we meet up and talk about this in person?" I wrote.

Dara: "No, it's not my job to educate you all."

Then a note: *Dara has left the conversation* from the operating system.

I looked up at the bulk storage bins of powdered herbs in the office. We had herbs for sleep, memory and skin plumping. I wished there was an herb to stop a fight. Or an herb to cure racism. The herbs were for the benefits we valued as a culture: beauty, productivity, calm. We are products of a system that trained us to be consumers, trained us to want to look good and feel good, not to inquire deeply into what is right.

When my ten-minute break was over, I was still trembling from the texts. I put my white apron back on to protect my white jeans and t-shirt. We were required to wear all white to give us a crisp, bright presence. It took a lot of awareness to not spill during all the juice related tasks. I took an order for a ginger beet immunity smoothie. I pushed the hi-speed blend button and the drink tornadoed out the top, splashing me with magenta froth. I had forgotten to put the lid on, consumed by the texts. Life gets messy.

I tried to be a safe sounding board for Dara's anger, but it was volcanic, and she started targeting me in our text messages. Being a Libra, fighting is hard for me. I don't want problems, I want harmony and fairness. "I want to see you get empowered," I told her, trying to be supportive. "How dare you tell a woman of color to get empowered, do you have any idea what I'm going through?" Dara's emotions were beyond my capacity to hold. I was seeing the deep wounds of racism she'd experienced. I didn't want to abandon her as a friend, but it felt like she had radicalized overnight, and I hadn't caught up. It hurt that she wasn't bringing me with her. This thing that was bigger then us was coming between us. I couldn't do enough to satisfy her expectations for what a white person should be doing to take responsibility for what my ancestors did. She was fierce in her anger towards me, almost like she was reveling in her power to shame me.

"Let's quit flipping who's the victim and who's the abuser, and figure out how to work together," I wrote Dara.

"Until you deal with your white supremacy all your supposed "healing" work is toxic," she responded.

In New York I had organized an alcohol-free party called The Softer Image. The idea was to create an altered state through group spiritual practice, decor, herbs and dancing. Dara had been a big supporter of the party and had helped do the decorations for the parties we'd thrown at the Dexter house in LA. I was trying to move forward and have another party without her, but she texted as the party approached.

"I want to come with my new crew of brown friends, can you comp us?"

"Of course." I hoped it would be a way to start a new chapter of understanding.

"I want it to be a safe space which means Calvin cannot be present."

"Well, it's Calvin's house. I can't tell him to not be in his own house." Calvin had been denying all of Dara's arguments: "Just because I don't have black friends doesn't mean I'm racist." His defensive, self-protective mindset couldn't listen and only made the argument worse. But, he was our roommate and friend. I didn't want to cut him out of my life because I didn't agree with his politics. I was pulled between them, wanting them to work it out. I figured Dara wouldn't be coming to the party.

The night of the party the air was dewy and jasmine scented. The patio was always party ready, I just hung some of the shimmery fabrics Dara and I had sourced downtown. The passion flowers stayed open, they wanted to come to the party, too. I was celebrating the end of my time at the Dexter house. Shane was returning to his room in a few days, and I was moving to a new sublet.

Canela had made a pot of rose and blue lotus cacao and served it to the group in mugs and shot glasses. Dee and Ruby DJ'd spiritual disco. We had a food altar of cut fruit, candles and crystals. About thirty people were there, some dancing, some sitting around the yard. The vibes were good. I felt my phone vibrate and it was a text from Calvin: "Dara's here and I don't feel safe. She texted me earlier she was going to spit in my face if I was at the party."

My body slammed into high gear with dread. I walked around looking for her. She was sitting at the patio table talking about how problematic Calvin's politics were. Fair enough, but this was his house.

She was dressed up in full queen splendor—a thin black ribbon around her neck, silk trench coat, black mini skirt, and slide platform sandals. She looked like the head of the Fashion Club. I tapped her on the shoulder to get her attention.

"Hey, I didn't think you were going to come?"

"But you said I could come."

"Well, I didn't think you'd come because of Calvin."

"I don't give a fuck."

I could feel my body gearing up to physically fight her and I really didn't want it to go that way. No one seemed to notice, the hum of conversation and disco beats continued.

"You have to leave. Now. I'm sorry."

"Lol. No. I. Don't. I have every right to be here just like everybody else does."

I'd never seen her face look like this before. There was a visible line of tension from her ears to her teeth. It looked like she was restraining herself from mauling me.

"Sorry but you have to go."

There was a hush to the conversations as people turned their attention to the fight that was brewing. The disco beats continued. "Sorry Dara, I don't want to do this, but I don't want to deal with this right now."

"I want my ash tray back." She grabbed the glass ashtray that looked like a faceted gem. It had been on the patio table since she lived there years ago. "And I want my Ram Dass books that are in the living room."

I was hoping some members of the Dolphin Pod would

emerge to try to mediate but only the closest people were watching what was happening. What was sad was that she hadn't triumphantly come with a new crew. She had come alone, and she'd have to leave alone. She started sobbing. "You guys are such. Fucking. Assholes." The people she'd been talking to at the table stood up to console her.

"Why don't you go get some tacos?" I said.

"Fine. I don't want to be at this lame party anyway." I opened the gate for her and the chime tinkled. "Do you have cash? Sorry I don't have any or I'd give it to you for tacos." That was the last thing I said to her for a long time.

No one texted on the Dolphin Pod chat after that. We all knew it was over. Seeing that eight people couldn't even coexist didn't give me much hope for the world learning to love one another. Our fight showed how polarized people are, even those of us who share the same values and want the same things, how stubborn we can get. "You don't understand." "No, you don't understand." "You are being insensitive." "No, you are being insensitive."

My dream of LA being a happy place without problems was shattered. My failure with the Dara situation made me doubt my communication and healing skills. Maybe the harmonious lifestyle I'd tried to cultivate was a mirage. My new sublet in Echo Park was quiet and lonely. I walked to and from work on Sunset ruminating on what it all meant. What did it mean to be white in this world? How to use my privilege to help make the world better? How to clean up the mess my ancestors made? The customers at the store seemed oblivious to the world outside their bubble, and I saw myself in them. We were all in "the matrix" we'd been raised in, taught to pursue comfort and buy stuff. I felt compassion but also a growing disgust. What would be needed for people to start waking up? For me it was losing a friend.

All relationships have a beginning, middle and end, and you learn things every step of the way. In the beginning Dara and I helped each other "become someone," by loving and validating each other. We propped each other up to create the version of self we wanted to perform in the world. In the end, when her love was taken away, I saw how dependent I'd become on her support. I had to learn to stand on my own. Maybe I let her down because I wasn't the woke healer I aspired to be. Maybe she had outgrown our codependent dynamic. Or both.

What really hurt was that Dara insisted I was not a good person. "Your healing work is toxic" really stung because I wanted to help, to be part of the solution. But walking home one night after work, I quit trying to deny it. I had always tried to be good, better even. What if I quit running away from bad and allowed myself to have some bad inside too, like everyone does? The Michael Jackson song started playing in my head, *I'm bad, I'm bad, you know it.* As I walked, I felt the heaviness from the fight lifting. I had missed Dara's actual point by getting triggered by how it hurt my ego. The neon signs on Sunset buzzed as I strutted under them. *Who's bad?*

The ego is our idea of who we are based on our memories and thoughts. It is a constructed idea of self that relies on the validation of the outer world; it is not the wellspring of spontaneous being. The artificial light turned eerie as I walked, the glowing gas station surreal. We lived in this paved and electrified Matrix world, like a sci-fi spiritual thriller, but it's real life. I felt my mind turning itself inside out. In giving up on being good, I didn't have to deny or resist Dara's critique. I could see that I too, was part of the problem, raised in a toxic matrix of programming and biases. If I was okay with being wrong, I could zoom out to see the whole problem and not get stuck in my own self.

For me, finding more freedom has been a process of undoing the constraints and limits of what I thought was acceptable or desirable in society. Re-wilding and un-learning was fun when it came to food, fashion, and sex, but awakening also means facing deeper problems. Dara showed me how my naivete about confronting the violence against people of color contributed to that violence persisting. It was like finding out I had been living with a disease, while contributing to it spreading. Nobody is all good; pretending we are is dishonest. Everyone has an ego they have to learn to keep in check. The situation helped me replace "being good" with just trying to be honest.

It was bold and brave of Dara to speak up and take a stand. If we are going to change the system we are going to have to get better at awakening, because I bet there are more matrixes we will face together. I hope we can grow to get over our personal reactions and figure out how to help each other. Maybe me and Dara will be able to be friends again someday, not because we're perfect but because all things eventually change.

16

Dark Ocean

At work we pour the expired juices down the drain. It's hard at first, but after a while you forget how precious the juice is. I would do juice art, layering the heaviest ones first, mango, coconut, and blue spirulina. Then I'd do the bottles of strawberry almond. As it all swirled down the drain it would marbleize and I would add dots of green juice and beet. That nightly release ritual, hundreds of dollars down the drain, taught me to not hold on.

It had been a record-breaking hot day and the shop wasn't as cold as usual. The heat lingered into the night. As I locked the door, hot wind blew in my face. Hot wind is the worst combination in Nature. Nobody likes the feeling of HOT WIND. Breezes used to be refreshing; now the climate has harshened, I thought, as I walked to my car. I rolled my one working window down and opened all the doors to release the built-up heat. You could have baked cookies in my car, it was so hot in there. Climate change was getting more real, I thought, as I drove away. The planet has a fever and may become unlivable in my lifetime. I made a snap decision to drive to the coast to cool off.

Turns out the crazy heat gave everyone the same idea. The Pacific Coast Highway was packed at 9pm on a Tuesday. It was 87 degrees, even with the sea breeze. I'd gotten to know Malibu since I first came with Ballet Surfer. Although it was haunted by heartbreak, it had also become a power spot that always offered me healing.

On the beach I passed a folding-chair family reunion and a couple carrying their flip flops as they walked on the shore. A little ways down, where I had some privacy, I left my shoes under a hazy streetlamp and jogged to the water. It was so dark I couldn't tell where the water stopped and the sky began. I got scared and second guessed my urge to swim. An undertow could whisk me away forever. Mother Nature asserts her control; no matter how advanced we get at overcoming her, she always has the upper hand. I wanted to trust her, to learn how to swim in the dark water.

I walked thigh deep into the chilly, bustling water. A wave crested and I dove under it, no time to hesitate. My body was shocked with cold, fear, and joy, all at once. Water is such an unfamiliar substance to be in, especially for someone from the desert. Something grabbed my ankle. Panic surged through me and I kicked my feet up, fearing there was a sea monster. Seaweed had gotten caught around my ankles. I tried to laugh it off but my body was surging with terror, what else was underwater that I couldn't see? My heart beat hard, I hoped my body heat didn't attract sharks. I dove under another peaking wave but it crashed right over me.

Underwater I had a dilated moment as I faced the abyss. This is it, I'm going to drown. I had dreamt it was the most poetic way to kill yourself, to just surrender to the sea. I felt some peace but also sadness. I had fantasized about checking out as an escape, when life got too hard. Who would find my white sneakers on the beach? My swim trunks would wash up with fang bites in them. Then I popped back up, smiling. I'm alive! I panted hard as my heartbeat slammed. I was shivering from the chilly water now and my survival instinct kicked in. I didn't want to die yet. Wow, this was a new side, the primal desire to survive. I hadn't felt so strong a YES in a long time. My arms went into superhero mode, and I got rolled under a few more times on my way back to the shore.

I laid on the sand dizzy, face up, spitting and sneezing salt water. At the Juice Shop we sold $4 ocean water shots you could drink. I had just drunk the equivalent of fifty of them. I had never been happier to be alive. Almost dying makes living feel triumphant. Nature had brought me back, shaken me awake.

I stood up and went to take a sip from the juice bottle I'd left by my shoes. It had expanded in the heat. I opened it and took a sip but it was rotten. I spit it out. I walked to the ocean and poured the juice back to its source, the source of all water, the source of life, completing its cycle. I felt fresh and salty, my nose clear and breathing deep. I didn't really want to leave the coast. It was like I had just had sex with the ocean and I wanted to cuddle, didn't want to rip away so quick. But I had to work the next day and figured I should get home while I was still cooled off.

I drove home barefoot feeling refreshed to the bone. Nature is the greatest healer. Maybe Nature's plan with climate change is to turn up the heat and bring us back into awareness of how much we need her. We are in a relationship with water and air, and we can't live in a world that's on fire. I reached for a cellophane wrapped raw chocolate bonbon from the Juice Shop, but it had melted. We are realizing that life isn't livable without the resources and temperateness we took for granted and polluted.

My car was eerily quiet in contrast to the extreme experience I had just had. As I drove in silence, I felt the sadness of how far removed our culture has become from Nature. I felt the contrast between the waves and the enclosed safety of the car. I always want to open windows and get fresh air, but so many places prefer air-conditioning. We've traded wildness for obedience as consumers. It felt strange to go from the wild waves to the rigid machinery and rules of the freeway. We sit in traffic to go to work to be able to afford things that make us feel almost as alive as swimming in the ocean. I could see downtown ahead, its buildings changing color with animated ads. Manufactured desires. More stuff for people to want. I felt so happy just being cold, salty, and barefoot. This was what I really wanted. Maybe I could move out to Malibu, but I probably couldn't afford it. Pristine Nature has become a rare commodity that gets more expensive every day.

The coolness in my bones was miraculous. I began to download insights from the Cosmos as I drove. My spiritual journey had started with the goal of living in harmony through yoga. I had thought I could always get the answers and achieve perfect health. But so much stress in my life had been about how to please myself, how to get the stuff I thought I needed. Spirituality had been another attempt to *get* something, What had really motivated me was fear. I was scared of life and was seeking secret ways to outsmart it. I thought I would make a calm, happy existence as an artist and healer in LA. But instead, I faced failures and disappointment, and my future had become increasingly unknown. Feeling the electric hum of my body and mind as I drove, I realized what I wanted wasn't security, but aliveness and spontaneity. To get into the dark ocean of the unknown. To brave the uncertainty. Life is never secure. There's too much randomness. And blessedness. I had no idea what was happening next in my life, and I felt at peace with it. There was joy in just being a body.

I slowed down as I hit a traffic jam. We inched along and I felt at peace. We came to a complete stop and I shifted my car into park. In the past, I would have been annoyed at the traffic. I would have thought about how over-populated the world has gotten and seen all the other humans as blocking me from getting where I needed to go. But that night, I felt compassion for the system that we are all trying to navigate. If there was a crash ahead, I hoped they were okay. I didn't feel an urgency to get anywhere. How had I gotten so out of sync, so restless? I rolled down the window to let in some hot night air and sat there in a spontaneous meditation. This was forever. I'd made it. I was finally here.

I turned on the radio and "Wouldn't It Be Nice" by The Beach Boys was playing. I started crying. It was such a clear message from God. This couldn't be an accident. This was one of the songs I used to listen to when I dreamt of LA. I cried as I listened to the bittersweet longing in the lyrics: *wouldn't it be nice to live together in the kind of world where we belong?* It was over so quick. Oldies are all under three minutes long. "Great oldies are back on K-Surf!" Some disco came on. I could hear the Universe guiding me through the music. Life is a party. I could see the humor in the unfolding illusions I had faced of all I thought I had to have to be happy. Happiness wasn't having everything I wanted, but dancing with the ups and downs.

Traffic picked up and the deep moment changed. I laughed at how quickly emotions can change. I flowed with the cars East. Then "Dreamweaver" came on, the gayest and sexiest song ever recorded. I blasted it as I got back up to high speed, wind blowing my hair sideways. I sang along. *Fly me high through starry skies, maybe to an astral plane, cross the highways of fantasy, help me to forget today's pain, oh dream weaver, I believe you can get me through the night!*

I could see the brake lights ahead again and was actually happy my ride home was being drawn out.

My cell phone lit up on the passenger seat. It was Pablo, the Painter from Portland. "I been thinking of you and still wanna make you some marbleized paper." We were clearly still psychically connected, he'd probably picked up on how strong I was vibing. I didn't feel like I needed to reply. It felt good to feel another human reaching out, but I felt totally complete in my car. Next, "Barbara Ann" came on, DJ God, giving me all the hits! The Love I'd been searching for was right here, listening to oldies, driving barefoot. I passed a billboard for Angelyne, the enigmatic LA pin-up girl. I was in love with life's craziness, the absurdity, the sadness, all of it.

Forty-five minutes later I made it past downtown, and home. I didn't want to turn the radio off because every song was still so good. "Crimson and Clover," was on, but I had work the next day. Every day is like the radio I thought, always a new song. I could finally let go and trust and I wasn't scared of ever running out of pleasure. This was the juice, the real nourishment. The juice that was already in us. Maybe this is what I had come to learn from the Angelenos. The Angels. I parked the Lexus next to a night blooming Datura bush. My time in LA was complete. I had gotten what I came for. I was fully hydrated.

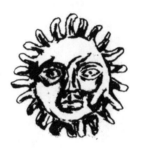

Gratitude

Cafes are a great place to write, meet people and overhear things. I want to thank the owners and staff of: Cafe de Leche, Valerie, Kaldi, Collage, Cabra, Abraco, Bakeri, Playground, McNally's & Bread Alone. Your foamy espresso hearts help me find the words for subtle feelings.

I am grateful to my friends, who are my muses, for their jokes and support. Especially to those I didn't write about, you are still a part of my story. There are some secrets I wanted to keep, and some stories I am saving for later.

Thanks to my family for supporting my non-linear path, even when it was unclear you encouraged me and felt like a pillar.

DJs Dirty Dave and Daddy Differently: I wrote to your weekly Dublab radio show, thanks for the trippy beats and banter.

To Ruby and the Numinous team! You were the perfect blend of supportive and honest with edits and advice. You made the process a joy and you were right, a book changes you, sometimes you have to grow before it's ready to come through.

To my lovers, our ephemeral moments filled me with life force and helped me learn about my attachments in Love and how I can be a more free and stable lover.

I didn't get to a destination, but to a point in my Self where I could embrace whatever I encountered with an open heart. This was not a realization I came to on my own, but the result of years of practice, study and encouragement from healers, movement teachers, authors and lineages of spiritual traditions like yoga, reiki and wicca. I hope that in sharing my path I contribute towards your reunion with the spark in yourself.

The entire writing process was filled with synchronicity. When I started realizing I could write about any experience, it made everything meaningful. I am still honing the ability to put words to feelings, but I want to thank Madelyn Kent and recommend her Sense Writing program.

Sense Writing helped me bypass the nervous static and blocks that had built up, damming my creativity, and finally reach the expression I'd been craving. In Sense Writing, you lay down and body map and do exercises to heal your brain and expand into new territory of the self. I want to keep exploring how creativity and healing are interconnected.